Y0-BYZ-235

ONE MILE
^AT ~A~ TIME

Cycling
through
Loss
to
Renewal

Dwight R. Smith

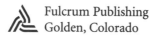

Fulcrum Publishing
Golden, Colorado

Text copyright © 2004 Dwight R. Smith

All rights reserved. No part of this book may be reproduced, stored in a retrieval system, or transmitted in any form or by any means, electronic, mechanical, photocopying, recording, or otherwise, without written permission from the publisher.

Library of Congress Cataloging-in-Publication Data
Smith, Dwight R.
  One mile at a time : cycling through loss to renewal / Dwight R. Smith.
    p. cm.
  ISBN 1-55591-461-6
  1. Smith, Dwight R.—Travel—United States. 2. Cyclists—United States—Biography. 3. Bicycle touring—United States. 4. United States—Description and travel. I. Title.
  GV1045.S55 2004
  796.6'092--dc22

                                                  2003020391

Printed in the United States of America
0 9 8 7 6 5 4 3 2 1

Editorial: Bob Baron, Daniel Forrest-Bank, Katie Raymond
Design: Patty Maher
Cover image: Jack Lenzo

Fulcrum Publishing
16100 Table Mountain Parkway, Suite 300
Golden, Colorado 80403
(800) 992-2908 • (303) 277-1623
www.fulcrum-books.com

*The journey was in memory of
Carol, Alan, and Mark.*

The book is for Yvonne.

Contents

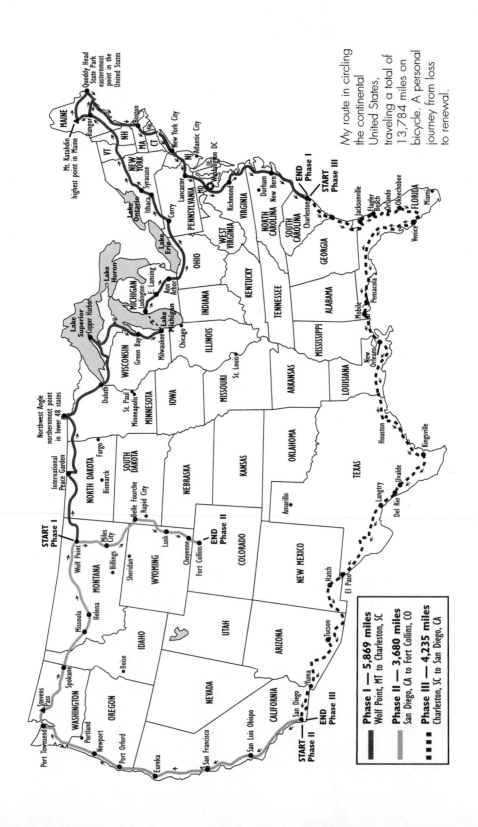

My route in circling the continental United States, traveling a total of 13,784 miles on bicycle. A personal journey from loss to renewal.

Phase I — 5,869 miles
Wolf Point, MT to Charleston, SC

Phase II — 3,680 miles
San Diego, CA to Fort Collins, CO

Phase III — 4,235 miles
Charleston, SC to San Diego, CA

Preface

This book tells the story of a 13,784-mile bicycle journey through thirty-four states. It is based on personal observations and facts recorded in ninety-four hours of taping, depicted in 2,500 photos, jotted in a notebook, and learned from research in libraries and other sources along the way and after I returned home. But did they accurately describe America and its people? Probably not. I am skeptical of politicians or tourists who go abroad for a few weeks, then return to describe a vast country and its people. They can't do it and neither can I.

What I can do is describe what I saw, heard, or otherwise discovered while biking around the perimeter of the United States. I might have encountered vastly different scenes and people had I traveled by auto or cycled on different roads. Which story would hold the truth about America and its people?

As a cyclist I experienced landscapes and people more intimately than if I had been isolated by two tons of glass and steel, comforted by heater or air conditioner, and distracted by radio or cell phone while hurtling along at seventy-five miles per hour. Weather influenced my descriptions more when riding a bicycle. On days bookended by gorgeous sunrises and spectacular sunsets, I was sometimes so stimulated by sights, sounds, and smells that my journaling became euphoric. When it was stifling hot, miserably humid, or cold, wet, and windy, my mood-driven outlook might plummet with my physical comfort.

Seeing America from the seat of a bicycle, however, offered benefits far outweighing disadvantages. I traveled slowly, stopped often, and frequently followed secondary roads. In campgrounds I met new friends who strolled over to inspect my bicycle and tent or to share a campfire and stories. At other times I spent a night, a weekend, or more, with impulsive folks attracted by my heavily loaded and travel-worn bicycle. A multitude of opportunities to learn the country and meet a rich diversity of people resulted from these chance encounters.

I purchased the bicycle and all equipment, and paid for film, tapes, and all other expenses; I was not financially obligated to anyone. No sponsor influenced where I rode or what I wrote. I asked no favors but received many from unbelievably generous strangers who received only my gratitude in return.

All events happened. All places exist. All names are of real people. In a few instances, when no good would be served and people might be harmed, I recorded what they did or said without mentioning their names.

This account, as honest as I can tell it, is about what I discovered in these incredibly diverse United States of America. I described photos, events, and conversations promptly on tape. This helped greatly to preserve accuracy over the long interval between their occurrence and writing this book.

Large cities often received scant attention as I competed with heavy traffic on narrow streets; I was more concerned with survival than getting acquainted. But I must admit to a preference for natural landscapes, other rural areas, and small towns. Those are the places I love most, know best, and wrote more about. Mostly, though, this is a story about people and relationships.

I began this solo journey in search of healing and returned home rich in new friendships, renewed faith, and improved physical and emotional health. At all four corners of the United States and along the paths connecting them, the kindness, concern, and warmth for a stranger were overwhelming. The hugeness of the American spirit touched me daily and I am the better for it.

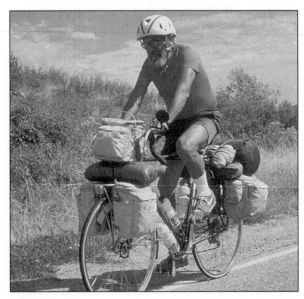

Hitting the road with my bike "Old Faithful" and all the gear (courtesy of Jim Osterberg)

Acknowledgments

No journey or book is truly a solo effort. A full list of those who contributed time, knowledge, skills, and great acts of kindness is too long to include. I hope it will be a small measure of thanks for those not mentioned by name to know that they have inspired me to more readily extend a helping hand to others.

The spiritual support and personal friendships of Fathers Tom McCormick, Leonard Urban, and Ron Weissbeck of John XXIII University Parish were there for me at critical times. Bert and Bernice Reid, and Jack and Yollanda Lebel, opened their homes for me when I returned to Fort Collins for medical care. Scores of folks befriended me as I pedaled the perimeter of our country and are mentioned throughout the book. To all of them, my gratitude.

Sandi Anderson earned special thanks for listening to ninety-four hours of taped narration, including outbursts of profanity, and transcribed it all into 1,900 pages of journal. She hung in there with me through good times and bad.

Paul Gentry, Ken Wilson, Peter and Darcy Molnar, thanks for your patience as we struggled with my computer-incompatibility.

It took a long time to overcome my preference for riding rather than writing. Libby James, who enjoys doing both, was the first to convince me I "had a book in me." The following reviewers helped me to say what I wanted to say: Jim Bailey, Billy Bush, Linda Cayot, George and Grace Dischinger, and Bill and Evie Weddel.

When words failed me utterly, Kevin Cook provided a machete to chop my way out of grammatical and stylistic jungles of my own creation. Jean Sutherland, despite a busy schedule, read my entire manuscript twice and e-mailed valuable suggestions during her travels in Virginia and Scotland. Others who generously helped with words and ideas include Frank Bostwick, Joe Friel, Larry Haise, Robert Leo Smith, and Ann Zwinger.

My son Gary and daughter, Sharon, supported me from the very beginning by saying, "Go for it, Dad," when others thought the idea to cycle around the United States was foolish. Their enthusiasm sustained me as I rode on my journey and struggled through the long book-writing project.

Yvonne, who came into my life nine years ago and soon learned about the "project" but had no idea how long it would dominate our lives, always had faith in me and the book. By reading and rereading the manuscript she got to know what was in my mind and heart, and her comments helped immensely to capture that on paper. I thank her for her love and patience.

Bob Baron at Fulcrum Publishing believed in my book. He and his staff skillfully brought my story to life.

CHAPTER ONE

The Journey Begins

Birds chattered outside my motel window, announcing dawn's arrival in Wolf Point, Montana. It was June 16, 1984, and I lay awake, thinking of Carol. Had she lived we would have celebrated her birthday today. Awake most of the night, I had tried counting sheep—in my case, bighorn sheep—but that didn't work. Instead, I visited and revisited memories of the thirty-nine years we had enjoyed together before her death fourteen months earlier. Finally, my thoughts shifted to when I would begin pedaling in a few hours and why I was doing it.

This personal journey had already begun as disconnected life-strands. During that sleepless night, I began to see how these strands were becoming interwoven, forming the thread that would pull me forward through dark times to a new beginning.

🚲 🚲 🚲

In 1965 my eighteen-year-old son, Alan, died in an auto accident south of Jackson Hole as he returned from climbing in the Grand Tetons of Wyoming. On that July day I had reviewed two of my graduate students' wildlife research projects in Yellowstone National Park. Early in the evening I pitched our tent and waited until Carol and our three other children settled in for the night. Then I drove a few miles to the Park's Grizzly Bear Study Headquarters, where an old friend, Dr. Frank Craighead, gave me an update on his bear studies as we drank coffee. The phone rang. Frank listened quietly for several minutes. "Dwight, someone wants to speak with you," Frank said as he handed me the phone.

"Dr. Smith?" Something in the solemn tone clutched my chest like a steel band.

"Yes?" I answered with a question.

"Do you have a son named Alan?" The band tightened.

Again I answered, "Yes?"

"We have been trying to reach you all day. I'm Sergeant Miller with the Wyoming State Patrol."

"I have to give you bad news," he said gently but with official brusqueness. "Your son was killed this morning in an auto accident in Hoback Canyon. I'm sorry, Dr. Smith."

I couldn't answer. I could hardly breathe. After a long silence, the sergeant continued, "Please put Dr. Craighead back on the phone."

I handed the phone to Frank, opened the back door, and walked down the tree-lined path to a pole fence where I leaned, gazing across a meadow drenched in pale moonlight. The scene was as cold and unreal as the voice on the phone.

Rejecting reality, my mind fled to a time when Alan was nine. For the previous three summers, he had traveled with me in the Idaho backcountry whenever it was feasible as I studied the life history and ecology of bighorn sheep. On a clearly remembered day, I was riding my saddle horse while leading four packhorses on a two-week trek into the Salmon River Wilderness

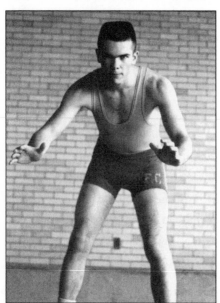

Alan was a mountain climber, an Eagle Scout, National Ski Patrol member, high school wrestler, and National Merit Scholar finalist. (Courtesy of Fort Collins High School)

Area to establish vegetation study plots. Alan rode behind the pack string on Blaze. We reached the Middle Fork of the Salmon River where I pulled up and called back, "Alan, I need to talk to you."

After working his horse around the nervous pack string, Alan asked, "What's up, Dad?"

"This water's swift," I warned. "If it knocks Blaze off her feet, grab the saddle horn and push yourself off on the upstream side. She'll be swimming and you might get kicked if you're downstream from her. Think you can do it?"

Even then Alan's gaze was direct, his words few. "Sure, Dad. I'll be okay."

I led the packhorses into the river and looked back. Without hesitation, Alan dug in his heels and yelled, "C'mon, Blaze!"

Alan forded the turbulent river with the same confident ability later displayed as he became a mountain climber, an Eagle Scout, then a National Ski Patrol member. In high school, he became a top-flight wrestler. He was also a National Merit Scholar finalist.

Other memories washed over me. Alan and I had skied, backpacked, climbed, and shared much. But we could have done much more together. I vowed to spend more time with my wife and surviving three children in the future.

A few weeks after Alan's death, however, those passionately declared intentions gave way to workaholic habits as I returned to the office nights and weekends to analyze data and write. Once, I isolated myself in a mountain cabin near the base of Pikes Peak in Colorado for three months to finish the dissertation required for a Ph.D. in ecology. Over the next few years, I progressed from assistant to associate to full professor of wildlife biology at Colorado State University.

⌚ ⌚ ⌚

Nine years after Alan's death, I was in my basement workroom one August afternoon, sanding a door that had been sticking. The phone rang and a voice asked, "Dwight Smith?"

"Yes?"

"Do you have a son named Mark?"

I remembered that tone of voice and lost control. "Don't you dare tell me my son has been killed," I shouted.

After a stunned silence the voice continued, softly, "I'm sorry."

Finally, I asked, "What happened?"

"A drunken driver careened across the median of I-25 north of Denver, hitting Mark head-on. Mark and his companion were killed instantly."

Randy Miller had worked with Mark in a Youth Conservation Corps camp all that summer and they had become close friends. After the camp closed, I contracted with the boys to paint our house. The job finished, seventeen-year-old Mark was taking Randy to his home north of Denver when the accident happened.

Numb, I hung up the phone and went back to sanding the door. A few minutes later Carol called down the stairway, "Dwight, what was the phone call?" Breaking from my trance, I ran up the stairs and held her tightly in my arms, unable to speak. She pulled back, horror in her eyes. "Has something happened to Mark?"

Carol was back in my arms again. Then, summoning her quiet strength and deep faith, she reached for my hand. "Let's go for a walk." Silently, we walked for blocks along elm-shaded Stover Street, trying to understand, to cope. Special memories of Mark welled up.

One recollection was especially poignant for me. I was living alone in a remote log cabin in the Collegiate Peaks mountain range in Colorado while filming a documentary on alpine ecology. Mark came in for a week of backpacking with me. He was a handsome, husky fourteen-year old, into bicycling and tennis, and already an avid reader of books on personal growth such as *Why Am I Afraid to Tell You Who I Am* by John Powell, Jesuit author and professor at Loyola University.

As we hiked together that week, I noticed that Mark tended to lose his sense of direction. I felt guilty for becoming so preoccupied with teaching and research that I'd not taught him the mountaineering skills Alan knew by this age. Early one afternoon I asked, "Mark, would you like to lead us back to our camp?"

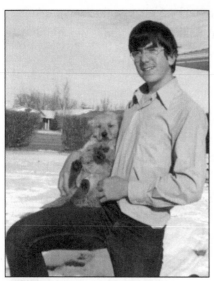

Mark too was a National Merit Scholar finalist. He and I were planning to hike the Rockies from Mexico to Canada.

Mark was hesitant. "Go ahead," I insisted. "You have followed me for three days. It's my turn to follow you."

Mark struck out ahead but was unusually quiet, often stopping to ask if we were headed in the right direction. "You're the leader," I'd say. We trudged on—and on. By late afternoon we were still a couple of hours from our camp. I didn't want to be hiking among those rugged 14,000-foot peaks after dark.

Finally I asked, "Mark, where do you think our camp is?"

"I'm not sure," Mark answered sharply. I looked at him closely for the first time.

"Well, we should get to camp before dark, so we need to cross this meadow and work our way up through that low saddle," I said, and pointed in a different direction than we had been hiking. "It's awfully easy to get turned around in these mountains, but you will do fine now," I assured him. "Would you still like to lead?"

"No," Mark snapped.

As we hiked along forest edges, across alpine meadows, over tundra-covered ridges, and skirted snowfields that never melt, Mark didn't say a word. We arrived in camp just before dark. After a silent supper, cooked on my backpack stove, I built a campfire in front of our tent, pulled up a log and sat, thinking about our day together. Mark dragged limbs and small logs to the edge of the flickering firelight, where he savagely chopped them into firewood lengths.

To break the silence, I remarked with a grin, "You have enough wood to last all night." Mark slammed his axe to the ground and flung himself on the far end of the log where he sat silently. After several failed attempts to open a conversation, I finally sat silently too.

For what seemed like ages we gazed into the fire, occasionally stirring it and adding more wood. Once after piling on wood, I returned to the log and sat down near Mark. He didn't move away. Minutes later, without warning, Mark threw his arms around me and choked, "I love you, Dad."

Soon we both had tears running down our cheeks.

I hadn't realized then that I had let Mark go through confusion, humiliation, and anger in trying to find his way home. I'd intended it as an important lesson in survival. Instead it was I who received the lesson. I must teach my son in more loving and understanding ways.

On the afternoon Mark died, police found a plan he had written as a high school project. It was for the two of us to hike the Rockies from Mexico to Canada. I had delayed the trip twice. Now the plan lay crumpled under broken shards of glass in our Fiat station wagon. Mark and I could have hiked the Continental Divide together if I had arranged to take the time. I promised myself once again that priorities must change.

A week after Mark's death, we received notice that he, like his older brother Alan, had become a National Merit Scholar finalist. Still later, his high school counselor sent us a plaque awarded to Mark when, as a junior, he had won his last tennis tournament.

Another nine years swept by. One afternoon as we were returning from a forty-mile bike ride, Carol suffered angina pains. Her doctor discovered problems in her heart, prescribed nitroglycerin pills for pain, and encouraged her to continue her active lifestyle. Later, though she was still biking thirteen miles daily to her job as a doctor's receptionist, cardiologists agreed she needed surgery to maintain the quality of life so important to her. Selfless as always, she insisted that before the surgery I go ahead with plans for a Grand Canyon backpacking trip with another professor, his wife, and nine graduate students during the university's spring break.

Carol went with me, stayed at a nearby lodge, and shared vicariously in the adventure. During the five days we hiked in the canyon, Carol read, wrote letters, and enjoyed short walks along the canyon's south rim. A few days after our return she entered a Denver hospital for open-heart surgery. My Carol never came home.

As the days of autumn shortened, they became the winter of my life. Our master bedroom was too large; our queen-size bed felt huge, out of proportion. I moved to a smaller bedroom and slept in a single bed. The loneliest spot of all was our family room with its large fireplace and broad sandstone hearth. From November through April it had been our ritual to light a fire after dinner and stoke it with aspen and lodgepole pine until we went to bed.

I remembered the once-a-week evenings when my ecology honors class met in this friendly place. We often munched apples in front of the fire while discussing the ecological concepts and environmental ethics championed in Aldo Leopold's *A Sand County Almanac* and Susan Flader's *Thinking Like a Mountain.* Carol enjoyed listening to these bright young men and women as she sat in the open kitchen alcove overlooking us. One

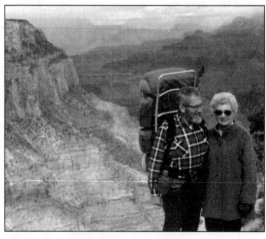

Before her open-heart surgery, Carol shared vicariously my Grand Canyon backpacking adventure. (Courtesy of Dr. Bruce Johnson)

winter she knit me a warm ski sweater while listening to our lively discussions. Always, she kept the coffeemaker going or had other hot drinks ready to serve.

Somehow, Carol knew when discussion was degenerating into argument or when we were wandering off the topic. At the perfect moment she would descend the five steps from kitchen to family room and announce a refreshment break.

I remember our quiet evenings alone even more poignantly. Carol would put her favorite cushion on the hearth, then sit, back to the fire, as she wrote letters or read. I would place a card table in front of the fire and prepare the next day's lecture or grade the last exam. Or I would sit in the Lazy Boy recliner, reading an ecology text to stay ahead of my students. Often we wouldn't exchange a word for hours as warmth from the crackling fire and Carol's nearness embraced me. On some evenings I would set two snifters of brandy on the hearth where they heated, gave off their enticing aroma, and later, warmed us before we went to bed. Although I was infinitely grateful for my two living children, if only Alan and Mark were still with us, life would have been complete.

After Carol's death my behavior began to change. For forty-five years I had often enjoyed a drink before dinner. Now, scarcely realizing it, I let one highball become two, then two stiff ones, then three. After finishing a third drink in front of the fireplace one evening and feeling lonely, frustrated, and sorry for myself, I hurled a heavy ashtray across the room, slicing a jagged groove across my writing desk and punching a hole in the wall.

The damage was insignificant. What was happening inside me was not. It frightened me. Sweat poured down my face as I sat, shaken. "Hell, I'm a better man than this," I exclaimed aloud. "This is no way to remember my loved ones."

After each death I had toughed it out, lecturing in front of my classes within a week after the funeral. This time ordinary toughness wasn't enough. I knew my life had to change. I unfolded the card table and drafted a letter to my dean at Colorado State University, notifying him of my intention to retire at summer's end.

My first night of retirement was one of tortured thoughts. I had slept fitfully, dreaming of Carol. In the dream she laid her hand on my leg and said in a tight voice, "Dwight, I need a pill." Sometimes Carol would forget to put her pill bottle beside the bed. If intense pain hit in the night, she often became so immobilized I would run to the bathroom for a nitroglycerin pill.

I awakened to find myself standing beside the bed, arm outstretched. I could still feel the tiny pill in my palm—and the warmth of Carol's hand on my leg. Disbelieving, I looked at my palm and at our bed. Both were empty.

It was three in the morning. I stayed up and put on the coffeepot. Later, I sipped coffee on our darkened patio and gazed at stars speckling the indigo sky as my mind went back—remembering.

⚲ ⚲ ⚲

Twelve years earlier, life as a professor had become routine, the numerous committee assignments downright frustrating. I finagled a filming assignment with Alan Landsburg Productions of Hollywood and took a leave from the university. Carol and Mark had stayed at home for five months while I lived alone in the Colorado mountains. I remembered what being apart had been like—for them and for me.

Ten years later restlessness resurfaced with visions of a colossal bicycle trip beginning to form. This time I would make it up to Carol by sharing the adventure with her. After all, we both commuted extensively by bike and enjoyed short bike trips together. I would take a year's leave without pay and using a motor home for support, we would alternate driving and bicycling around North America. A compulsive planner, I outlined a schedule that would take us 15,000 miles around the perimeter of the United States in forty-eight weeks. Just right for a year's leave—with a little time to spare. I would bankroll the adventure with a loan and worry about paying it off when I returned to the university to finish my career.

But faculty staffing was short, making it awkward to ask for a year's leave, and Mark was still in junior high. We would have to wait a few years.

⚲ ⚲ ⚲

By the time the coffee was gone and golden rays of dawn invaded the starlit sky, I had made two major decisions. Chilled, I pulled on my sweater, brought out a pad of writing paper, and began outlining plans.

The notion of seeing America up close still appealed to me. In keeping with habits of a lifetime, I would seek healing through vigorous exercise, preferring physical pain to emotional anguish. I decided to bike around the United States alone, dedicating the journey to Carol and the two sons I had lost. I would begin near the Canadian border at Wolf Point, Montana, and ride clockwise around the perimeter.

I also decided that morning to learn to fly. Before World War II, one of my friends at the University of Idaho had taken flying lessons. Though it was illegal to fly with a student pilot, I had pitched in $1.50 an hour to share his $3.00-an-hour, three-bounce landings. I was hooked. The day after Pearl Harbor, I tried to enlist in the Army Air Force but failed the eyesight test. Flying would have to wait. Over the years, I went to war, finished college, worked, and raised a family, but never found time or money for flying lessons. Now I would fulfill a forty-four-year dream.

The next eight months were hectic. Flight training. Bicycle trip planning. Preparations. My emptiness began to diminish, filled by the exhilaration of new challenges.

My ancient ten-speed Schwinn would never make a long tour. After reading bicycling books, magazines, and manuals, and consulting experienced bicyclists, I selected a Specialized Expedition eighteen-speed touring bike, a choice I never regretted. Later, after riding a few hundred miles, I assigned the bike the female gender and an affectionate name, Old Faithful.

My first experience with her was a forty-five-mile ride to visit bike-touring guru Hartley Alley in Boulder. Hartley had toured widely in the United States, British Isles, Europe, and the Orient. He also manufactured cycling gear in his Touring Cyclist shop. I returned with four panniers, a handlebar bag, tools, accessories, and the benefit of Hartley's experiences in defensive bike riding. I was skeptical, however, about one bit of advice.

"When you get in a tight spot on narrow roads," Hartley cautioned, "don't let motorists force you off the road. Signal, then move smartly to the center of the lane. Don't hesitate or they won't realize what you're doing. You may be the target of profanity and obscene gestures but they won't hit you, if for no better reason than keeping your blood and guts off their windshield."

Months later, after being run off the road in Michigan and Maine and tumbling ass over teakettle into the ditch both times, I appreciated the wisdom of Hartley's words and began claiming the traffic lane. Enduring profanity and the finger was the lesser price to pay.

I considered maintenance and repair needs. For the bicycle, I bought standard bicycle tools, a spare tube and tire, extra chain links and wheel spokes, a bike lock, and a waterproof bicycle cover. For myself, I assembled medications for headaches, chafing, sunburn, and blisters.

My plans to fully record the journey required more equipment. I purchased a Pentax camera with a 28 to 80mm zoom lens and a tape recorder with lapel mike to attach under my chin on a T-shirt or jacket. To protect sensitive items, I cut a block of Styrofoam to fill the interior compartment of the handlebar bag and carved spaces for camera, tape recorder, film, tapes, and batteries.

Planning to camp whenever possible, I packed a tent, sleeping bag, and foam pad. My wardrobe, other than a pair of polyester slacks, two short-sleeve shirts, a light jacket, and a pair of leather moccasins, was strictly biking gear— shorts, shirts, shoes, gloves, sweats, Gortex rain gear, and a helmet. Heeding repeated warnings about long dry stretches, I attached a third bottle mount to the frame and purchased three sixteen-ounce water bottles. In all, I carried three pints of water. Not enough, I realized later in desolate parts of the Desert Southwest. Still, I'd added sixty-one pounds of equipment and supplies to my twenty-four-pound bike. At this point I abandoned plans to carry equipment or groceries for camp cooking. Instead, energy bars, snacks, and fresh fruit would fuel me from one restaurant to the next.

In the first weeks of the journey, I rearranged gear almost daily. Weight distribution, not only side to side but fore and aft, was critical to safe and comfortable touring. My conclusion was that 40 percent of the weight in front and 60 percent in back worked best. Eventually I could tell if a pair of shorts or socks was in the wrong compartment when I started riding in the morning. Well, perhaps that's a slight exaggeration!

Another need was to plan an itinerary. One part of me wanted just to be a free spirit. Fly to Wolf Point, Montana, climb on the bike, and start pedaling east. Another, more rational part acknowledged my nearly sixty-three years and cautioned that such action could lead to disaster instead of a circle around the United States.

Fortunately my thirty-one-year association with graduate students had generated a network scattered throughout the United States. They were indispensable in selecting routes to travel and places to stay. Equally important was their knowledge of natural landscapes and their plant and animal inhabitants. Often they knew of cultural and historical treasures that would enrich my journey.

Sharon, our second child, and sixteen months younger than Alan, graciously offered to handle any business or legal matters during my sojourn, so I provided her with my power of attorney. She didn't know at the time that a whole shelf in her home would be needed to store books and other literature I would collect along the way.

To keep in touch with family and friends, I provided them with general delivery addresses in sixteen towns where I would pick up mail along my route. Finally, I arranged with my neighbor in Fort Collins, Sandi Anderson, to transcribe the dictation-filled tapes I would mail.

While all these preparations were underway, friends often asked if I had trained for the ride. No, I admitted, but a bicycle had been my principal commuting vehicle, and I had logged more than 40,000 miles in the past twenty-five years. I would have to toughen up for distance cycling with on-the-job training.

Just when I thought everything was in order and I could relax until departing for Wolf Point, my family doctor proposed that it would be interesting to use my body for a mini research project. Some friends at Colorado State University assembled a team, including a cardiologist, a doctor of sports medicine, and an exercise physiologist, that directed a grueling sequence of exercise stress tests, plus strength, endurance, and flexibility measurements during my last two weeks in Fort Collins. They also conducted body fat tests, a complete blood chemistry profile, pulmonary function evaluations, and took "core samples" for a thigh-muscle biopsy. These tests would be repeated after my ride to learn the effects of sustained high-level exercise on my senior citizen body. Many nights I dragged home from the University Human Performance Lab with tongue hanging out, thinking, "You damned fool. Why are you doing this to yourself?"

The week before leaving home, I felt like the Bengali poet Rabindranath Tagore: "The song that I came to sing remains unsung to this day. I have spent my days in stringing and in unstringing my instrument. The time has not come true, the words have not been rightly set; only there is the agony of wishing in my heart."

Edgy and irritable, I didn't sleep well. The urge to fly to begin my long-planned bicycle trek was upon me.

For several mornings I called Denver Flight Service only to hear reports of thunderheads, ground fog, or cold fronts. Finally the forecast was more encouraging: "Except for ground fog, you should have good VFR [Visual Flight Rules] conditions tomorrow morning."

At Fort Collins Airport my daughter, Sharon, and son Gary helped dismantle the bike and cram it into the luggage compartment. Sharon, an occupational therapist and a pilot, had flown a small plane from her home in Aspen, which she shared with her husband, Lou, and two small children, Dustin and Kari. Lou, a veterinarian, owned a small- and large-animal clinic there.

Gary had taken a commercial flight from Atlanta where he lived with his wife, LaVerne. Gary was employed by Diversified Business Investments, involved in listing and selling small businesses in and around Atlanta. Our third child, he was four years older than Mark.

I was grateful they had come to share in the beginning of my adventure.

The next morning my adrenalin was pumping as I anticipated my first major flight since earning a pilot's license a few weeks before. My thoughts moved to the time when I'd missed my destination on a cross-country flight. When I finally found the field there were only five minutes of fuel in the tanks. However, today's crisp air, gentle breeze, and bright blue sky instilled confidence, not doubts. Sharon sat up front as navigator. Gary shared the backseat with four fully packed panniers, a handlebar bag, rolled-up tent, sleeping bag, foam pad, and three water bottles.

Coaxing the heavy-laden, four-place Cessna 172 off the short runway in Fort Collins and into the radiant dawn, I turned to a heading of north. Denver Flight Service was right. Ground fog lay peacefully beneath us, looking like rumpled bedspreads glistening in the morning sun.

Two hundred and fifty miles of Colorado mountains and Wyoming desert slipped quickly behind us before I landed in Gillette. We stopped for breakfast and a visit to the bathroom for us, then 100-octane low-lead and drained fuel petcocks for the plane. We all felt better as we continued north.

No one was at the tiny airport when we landed in Wolf Point, Montana. I found a phone and called a motel to ask about a room and transportation into town. "Sure, I've got a van that will haul your bicycle and gear," said the motel owner. "You're riding where? Well, I'll be!" A gentle breeze moderated the sun's warmth as we reassembled the bike. I began to relax.

ڳڳ ڳڳ ڳڳ

At dawn on June 16, Carol's birthday, I mounted Old Faithful and spun past the city limits of Wolf Point, turned east on State Highway 2, and began the first mile of what would become a 13,784-mile trek. Sharon and Gary had left earlier for the airport where we planned to meet for goodbyes before Sharon full-throttled into the early morning sky. Bike tires hummed as first-day thoughts spilled into the tape recorder: "Rains dotted the Montana landscape during the night, leaving moist asphalt and fresh smells of Missouri River bottomland to tell the story. I wonder what adventures lie ahead."

Suddenly, the feeling that I had pedaled past the airport turnoff interrupted my reverie. I started flagging cars to find out if I'd gone too far. Several sped past my waving arms before one stopped. It was Gary, looking for me.

"You passed the airport road, Dad," Gary said with a smile, "but it's two miles off the highway and deeply graveled. Sharon wants to take off before the air gets hot and bumpy. She'll understand if you don't ride back." Numbly agreeing, I hugged Gary, mumbled some awkward words, and rolled eastward, alone with my thoughts.

After two hours I stopped at Lee's Coffee Shop in Poplar. I was already feeling pain in my right knee and elbow. My hands tingled and my left foot felt a little numb. I'd pedaled only 12.6 miles.

At noon I checked in at the Elkhorn Motel in Culbertson, showered, and surveyed my body for physical damage. Sore toes, diagnosed as toenails too long, and exhaustion, diagnosed as training too short, were quickly treated by wielding toenail clippers and collapsing across the bed.

Soon rejuvenated, I celebrated in my room with a small flask of vodka I had slipped into a pannier for the occasion. Orange Crush from the motel's soft drink machine created a bland screwdriver. It would take time to gather enough courage to walk into a Montana bar in bicycling shorts and drink with the cowboys. After dinner at the Lamplight Inn, I was ready for bed again.

Still, fifty-eight miles by noon of the first day wasn't bad!

CHAPTER TWO

Northern Prairies

On a tranquil summer day, the green of the prairie seems like a vast ocean, dominated by grass in such dense stands that only the mosaic of cloud shadows breaks the endless serenity of the view.

—David F. Costello,
The Prairie World

Awake at sunrise, I anticipated Sunday on the prairie and felt serene for the first time in weeks. At six o'clock, I pedaled north toward Froid, Montana, leaving the Missouri River where it turned to meander southeast to the Mississippi.

Climbing steadily, I noticed cottonwoods and oaks in the ravines. Fields surrounded by flowering roses and dotted with thickets of wild plum told me this was excellent pheasant habitat. Two-syllable notes from a cock pheasant confirmed my judgment while hen pheasants responded to the passion in his calls. Melodious songs of meadowlarks atop fence posts and bubbling lyrics of bobolinks flitting above the prairie grasses blended into a Sunday morning hymn.

The three-mile climb out of the Missouri River Valley took a half hour. Despite cool headwinds, sweat trickled down my arms and body and slid off my nose. If this was so hard, what of the miles ahead?

🚲 🚲 🚲

Two questions most asked before I left home had been: "Are you in condition to complete the journey?" And, "Won't the loneliness do you in?" I had answered, almost flippantly, that I wasn't concerned. Since my early teens, I'd worked hard and had often been alone. I hoped my background would be adequate preparation for the grueling days ahead.

Reared on hardscrabble ranches and in the forests of northern Idaho, I had grown up during the Great Depression. From age ten I tended livestock, milked cows, and sawed and split firewood before and after school. Beginning before my thirteenth birthday, and for the next five years, I drove a team of horses to plow, disc, and harrow the soil before planting crops each spring. Summer meant haying and cultivating row crops. Grain and potato harvest filled the days of autumn.

Other work finished, I'd go to a corner of our ranch to cut brush and trees with an ax and saw, then dig around the roots with a "grub hoe" so my team of horses could yank them out. The purpose of this effort was to carve a new field from the scrubby forest.

From high school graduation in 1938 until completion of a third college degree in 1971, my life was stop-and-go academia. Interspersed through these years were stints as a lumberjack in the Northwest, truck driver in the Midwest, construction worker in Alaska and Idaho, and combat infantryman in the Aleutians and Europe. Along the way, my professional career developed with titles of wildlife biologist, area game manager, extension specialist, research scientist, and university professor.

I studied bighorn sheep for four years, including one entire winter in the Idaho Primitive Area, now the Frank Church Wilderness Area. Carol and I lived fifty miles from the nearest open road with our first two children, five-year-old Alan and three-year-old Sharon. Twice monthly I snowshoed a fifty-mile circuit along treacherous mountain trails. Further research on bighorn sheep, conducted from a high-country tent camp far from any road, occupied a full summer. Whitewater rafting and horse packing trips lasted from a week to six weeks each. Later, I spent five months working and living alone in a log cabin high in the Colorado Rockies.

Downhill and cross-country skiing, mountain climbing, backpack camping, and big game hunting were favorite recreational activities for me. When nearly forty, I started jogging and at fifty began running in "age-class" competitions. A marathon in Winnipeg, Manitoba, was a challenge at age sixty.

"Yes," I congratulated myself, "I'm used to being alone and I'm in great shape. I'll circle these United States come hell or high water." As it turned out, there was more hell and high water than expected—and I failed to figure in headwinds!

🚲 🚲 🚲

Breakfast business was booming at the cafe in Froid. The one-armed owner-cook-waiter was neat and amazingly dexterous as he served a superb breakfast. A garrulous customer talked about an incident at the other restaurant in town. Some biologists from nearby Medicine Lake Wildlife Refuge were having coffee while talking about their studies of the endangered whooping crane. The waitress put her coffeepot down in disgust and asked, "If they're so dangerous, why are you wasting taxpayers' money to study them? Why don't you just shoot the damn things?"

After breakfast I enjoyed bright sunlight and invigorating air while riding to a small white church at the upper edge of Froid. A convert to the Catholic faith, I usually attended church but was not concerned about going to hell in a handbasket if I missed. This morning, though, I strongly felt the need to receive communion, perhaps as a blessing for my trip.

Early for mass, I sat on a grassy knoll near the parking lot and waited. Parishioners, many arriving in pickups, exchanged neighborly greetings, weather commentaries, crop reports. A few were Native Americans but for the most part the swarthy complexions resulted from years of wind and pollution-free sunlight. Many glanced at my touring bike. Others smiled and called, "Good morning!"

Later, in church, I moved forward with others to receive communion, then returned to my seat and prayed. I felt good, but no more uplifted than earlier when I had watched and listened as this prairie community gathered for worship. Perhaps I had attended church before walking in the door.

In Antelope the locals warned that I couldn't bike across four miles of fresh asphalt just ahead, so Steve Martin, a federal biologist, hauled me and Old Faithful across in his pickup. Fewer than a hundred miles into the trip, and I had already suffered the indignity of hitching a ride!

After leaving a motel in Plentywood the next morning, I rode to Plentywood Electric where Greg Nielsen repaired my tape recorder, replaced the nonfunctioning toggle switch, and welded a broken toe clip. He refused pay. "Your money's no good here. Anyone with guts enough to undertake a trip like that isn't going to pay." At Petersen's Hardware, Jerry Iversen lent tools and his workbench for me to repair the odometer. All these repairs after only three days on the road! But I was grateful for the friendly generosity of Greg and Jerry.

ᚣᚣᚣ   ᚣᚣᚣ   ᚣᚣᚣ

Lakes and ponds dotted the landscape as I entered North Dakota. Watching the soft glow of the setting sun, I could hardly imagine that these pastoral scenes evolved through violent acts of nature. Since the Pleistocene epoch more than a million years ago, there have been four major ice advances and retreats. Great hunks of ice imbedded in the glacial debris melted, creating thousands of small basins that filled with water and became ponds in what we call the "pothole country" today. Between glacial periods, roaring winds carved the present landscape.

Next morning I moved steadily along, enjoying the light green of fields and soft tones of earth and stone. Passing contented cows and ponds surrounded by cattails and singing blackbirds, I imagined the history of this changing land. First oceans and marine creatures. Then lush plants and dinosaurs followed by eons of icy desolation and later, grasslands, bison, and humans. Only the last few seconds, as measured in evolutionary time, brought highways, towns, and agribusiness to displace the sea of prairie grasses.

Just before Larson, a cemetery across the road from a simple white church told stories on stone. It was only a half acre of grass, fringed sage, a few lilacs, and two short rows of large solid headstones. I leaned my bicycle against the headstone of Otto Evanson (March 16, 1864–October 25, 1947). Next to Otto is his wife, Eline, who died in 1938. Her headstone reads, "Mother, she is at rest in heaven." Tender sentiment in the midst of the harsh depression and dust bowl years.

Lilacs flanked two other stones: "Casper Larsen, corporal, 16th Cavalry, Spanish-American War, 1869–1953; Olava Larsen, 1883–1923." Back in the lilacs another stone read, "Curtis Larsen, 1907–1919." Curtis was born when his war-veteran father was thirty-eight and his mother twenty-four. He died at age twelve. Four years later his mother died. Still nursing my own sense of loss, I wondered if his father lived his final thirty years as a widower.

Two hundred yards east of the cemetery, a road led to the town of Larson. Two signs advertised Border Club—Live Entertainment and Triangle

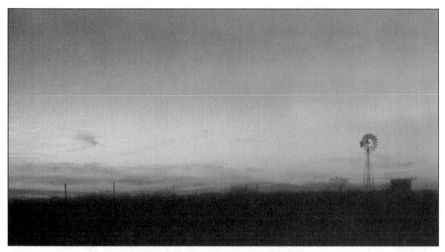

Windmills punctuate the landscape in North Dakota. They bring water to the surface for crops, livestock, and people.

Steakhouse—Cocktails. My mind wandered to a book I had read in high school. In Rolvaag's *Giants in the Earth,* the bible was quoted to describe life on the prairies more than a century ago: "There were giants in the earth in those days; and also after that, when the sons of God came in unto the daughters of men, and they bear children to them, the same became mighty men which were of old, men of renown" (Genesis 6:4).

How does one measure the mightiness of men? Of women? Were the Hansons, Larsens, Evansons, and others true "giants in the earth"? Or is that nostalgic nonsense? Are today's patrons of the Border Club and Triangle Steakhouse of equal moral stature? I didn't stop at the Border Club or the Triangle Steakhouse, nor did I talk to anyone in the town of Larson. It was just as well. I needed heroes—if only in my dreams.

East from Columbus, the roadsides were clean and grass-covered. Neatly mowed farm lanes bordered by American elms, North Dakota's state tree, led to sturdy, well-maintained white houses and red barns. Wild prairie roses, the state flower, grew in clumps or climbed fence posts. Twining stems displayed their delicate pink blossoms.

By midafternoon the sun was hot and I was dry. Leaving my bike beside a tree, I walked down a lane and circled a farmhouse in search of someone to ask for water. Three dogs uncoiled from the back steps. One challenged my bare legs with bared teeth. The back door opened and a tall, lean farmer in bib overalls and with only one visible tooth silently surveyed the ruckus as his wife and son peered over his shoulder. To explain my helmet, biking shorts, and purpose, I offered, "Left my bicycle at your entrance. Could I fill my water bottles, please?"

The farmer's eyes narrowed suspiciously, "I thought someone was snooping around."

"I knew you might wonder, so I came around to let you know who I am."

"I still don't know who you are," he said and closed the door. Though still thirsty, at least I didn't become dog food!

ڵ ڵ ڵ

I walked into the Paragon Restaurant in Mohall where two young men asked me to join them for breakfast. John Hauptman was a petroleum land-man for Intermountain Leasing, an oil company subsidiary. Jim Reid was his associate. Their jobs included arranging for exploration and drilling leases on private and public lands. After John picked up the tab, he said they would like to take me to dinner that evening in nearby Sherwood.

At the Northern Lights Restaurant that evening, we enjoyed authentic Norwegian torsk (codfish with sugar added), steamed and served with hot butter and lemon. Afterward John, Jim, and I talked about oil companies, prairie country, and people.

"The first successful oil well in North Dakota," John told me, "was drilled near the town of Tioga in 1951. In the early sixties, Oklahoma and Texas oil companies began buying underground rights."

"Although the energy resources are potentially very valuable, landowners in this area cherish their independence," Jim explained. "They don't want outsiders, whether private industry or government agencies, to dictate what they do with their land."

John agreed. "I will contact a landowner about leasing mineral rights on his land. Months pass. We may see each other in stores, restaurants, or bars. Yet he never mentions the unfinished business of leases. It takes about six months from planting to harvesting a crop. It often takes a farmer as long to respond to a leasing offer."

"Farmers are not trying to 'outstrategize' the oil company," Jim added. "They simply will not rush into such an important decision."

Our conversation expanded my understanding of this land. Grass, pot-holes, and ducks always symbolized the prairie for me. I had never considered the "black gold" beneath the grassland sea.

Long before daybreak the next morning, I awoke to howling wind and pouring rain. After an hour of looking at the sky, putting on rain gear, looking at the sky, and taking off rain gear, I finally settled on biking shorts and T-shirt. "C'mon, a little rain won't hurt you," I chided myself.

My courage was rewarded with bird songs and the sweet aroma of wet earth. A spectacular sunrise greeted me through rising mist. A huge sign covering the end of a barn proclaimed, "Glory to God." This seemed ostentatious, but the theology suited the mood and setting. Glory, indeed!

As I climbed into the Turtle Mountains, slanting rain began to pelt the road and me. Winds hurled gravel, dust, and pieces of tar paper from a construction site across the road. One violent gust nearly threw me over an embankment. I was happy to reach Lake Metigoshe State Park, be off the bicycle and snug in my tent, even without dinner. This was my longest day in the first week—more than seventy-two miles.

I felt stiff in the morning, but a brisk ride around the lake loosened me up and whetted my appetite for breakfast at Turtle Mountain Lodge. The owner's wife asked if she could call a local newspaper reporter. "Thank you, no," I replied. "This is a personal journey."

Over coffee I learned that Turtle Mountains describes a region of rolling, forested hills that include Lake Metigoshe and extend northward into Manitoba. Many lakes and ponds provide human recreation and wildlife habitat. Lake Metigoshe, with seventy-six miles of shoreline, dominates the state park. Metigoshe stems from the Indian word *Met-i-go-she-sah-hig-gun,* meaning "the clear water surrounded by oaks."

Nearing International Peace Garden at the Canadian border, I startled a shy white-tailed doe beside the road. The deer dashed alongside for a hundred yards, striding gracefully at my speed of twenty-four miles an hour, before leaving me for the solitude of the forest.

I pitched my tent in the campground, then rode around the U.S. and Canadian sections of the Peace Garden. Later, I paused at the sunken garden. A few years ago, Carol and I had stood here, entranced by the tranquil scene. This time, I photographed the panorama of flowers and manicured shrubs as

I had then. Turning, I saw a penny and picked it up. I thought, "Well, Carol, I beat you to that one." She was adept at finding coins wherever she went and had saved them for our grandchildren. For a moment her hand seemed to be in mine as I walked back to the bicycle.

After a refreshing shower in a restroom near my tent, I passed two couples playing cards on a picnic table. "Where are you camped?" one woman asked.

"Over in that tent."

They broke into laughter. "That little blue one? We thought it was too small for a grown-up. We saw the bicycle chained nearby and figured a little kid must have ridden from town to go camping all by himself. It looked so cute."

The couples, from North Carolina, were on a leisurely trip to Alaska. Wesley Winstead's wife, Mildred, took me aside and explained that Wesley had had a heart attack two years before in 1982 and the prognosis wasn't good. "But I'm going to see that we do everything possible in the time we still have," Mildred confided.

I recalled the words a Catholic priest friend wrote a few days after Carol's death: "I have been touched deeply by both of your lives. I realize how closely your lives were intertwined and know the letting go is especially hard because of your love and the hopes you had of sharing so much more." It was too late for me to turn back the clock, but I was glad the Winsteads were grasping the moment.

Later I slid into my sleeping bag and zipped up the tent. The night's entertainment featured an inchworm measuring the mosquito netting just above my

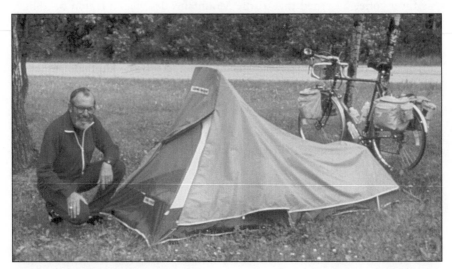

The tent is small but serves its purpose.

nose. Music and laughter wafted on fragrant air from across a wooded glen where a wedding party was in progress.

Drowsily, I thought of Carol as a fresh breeze blew across my face and a dazzling array of stars backlit the inchworm. Sleep came quickly.

The next morning the Winsteads and Bowes saw me hanging tent and gear up to dry and called, "Come over for breakfast!" Steaming coffee washed down homemade bread, pear preserves, and doughnuts as we chatted about plans for the future. Anticipation for the new day transcended last night's wistful reflections. What a way to jump-start a Sunday morning!

After attending nondenominational services at the Peace Garden Chapel, I headed south on State Highway 281, then turned east through Dunseith. A sign advised that Rugby, the geographical center of North America, was thirty-two miles to the south. I was truly in the heartland.

After a night in the Rolla Motel, I awoke with considerable pain in my ankle. It seemed a good morning to do my laundry before heading out of town. By midmorning my ankle began to swell spectacularly and throb for no apparent reason. A nurse in the Rolla Clinic recommended aspirin and rest. She then wrapped it with an elastic bandage.

I called Sharon to get some sympathy. "Are you ankling, Dad?" she asked. "Am I *what?*"

"Ankling. You rotate or flex your ankles with each stroke of the pedal. That might help prevent swelling and stiffness."

Fine time to find out, I thought, as I lay on the motel bed with my ankle elevated on an ice pack. The pain lessened after a couple of hours. While resting I read about the local William Langer Tool Bearing Plant operated by Bulova Watch Company. To test my ankle before serious pedaling, I rode out of town a few miles to visit it.

Supervisor Daniel Vining took me through the plant. Jewel bearings used in guidance systems and other military devices are the company's main products. The bearings are so small that "several could get lost under your fingernail," he told me. Chippewa Indians, mostly women from Turtle Mountain Reservation, make up a large part of the workforce.

"Management ideas have changed since the plant opened in 1953," Vining explained. "At that time men were thought to have more mechanical aptitude and more ability for inspection and supervisory positions. Women, it was thought, had more patience for repetitive tasks on the assembly line. Experience has shown that such attributes are not necessarily gender linked. Now men often work on production lines and several women are in supervisory positions."

Early the next morning I glided smoothly out of Rolla as I thought of Thomas Merton, the sensitive Trappist monk who wrote, "The most wonderful moment of the day is that when creation in its innocence asks permission to 'be' once again as it did on the first morning that ever was."

By 6:15 A.M. I'd delighted in the shyly emerging glory of the sunrise and ridden more than eight miles. Cool breezes ruffled my beard. Prairie fragrances intoxicated my senses. Pairs of mallards, mixed with a few pintails and green-winged teal, romanced with delightful abandon in the rich prairie marshes.

But marshes are more than sunrises, caressing breezes, and wild romances. Gazing across the magnificent wetlands, I remembered a study by my friend, David Costello. Dave listed more than 1,100 plant and animal species living in and around a prairie pond smaller than an acre. I wondered how many motorists notice this abundance while hurtling along State Highway 5 at seventy-five-plus miles per hour. Do they know how wetlands store water to reduce flood damage and recharge underground aquifers with water for future needs? Do they understand that while crops, coal, and oil serve human needs other important values result when a prairie is allowed just to *be?* Probably not, or public policy wouldn't be to drain, plow, plant, and pave wetlands at the rate of nearly a half-million acres a year.

Later I paused to photograph a collage of colors—dark-green windbreaks, light-green spring wheat, golden sunflowers, black summer-fallowed soil, blue sky, and striated white clouds.

I ground out sixty-four miles by noon, arriving in Langdon in a drenching thunderstorm. At the Nodak Motel, I promised to wipe off the tires and place newspapers under the wheels before the woman in the office would allow my bicycle in the room.

Later, when I asked for a lightbulb to replace a burned-out one, her husband refused. "If I let you change it," he growled, "you'll hurt yourself and sue us." When he marched into the room and saw my bike, he exploded. I interrupted his tirade by grabbing the bicycle and heading out the door. When he realized I was going into the downpour, he spluttered something about damages by vandalistic guests, then relented with, "Well, since you're here, I guess you can stay."

Months later my bike and I received royal treatment in plush resorts, at Howard Johnson's in Boston, and at the Waldorf-Astoria in Manhattan. Even at seventeen dollars a night, Ma and Pa motels aren't always a bargain.

                                        d̳ d̳ d̳

I leaned Old Faithful against the bridge railing and photographed her waiting to carry me across the Red River into Minnesota. The Red flooded in 1979 with disastrous results to Grand Forks a hundred miles downstream and to small communities and farmland along the way. Marshes and ponds, serving as nature's sponges, would likely have absorbed enough surging water to avert much of the damage if they hadn't been drained, plowed, and replaced by paved developments.

A familiar scene as I approached Salol included a couple dozen homes, a church, the Farmer's Union Cooperative Association, and a grain elevator. In North Dakota and northwestern Minnesota, the first evidence of an upcoming town is the ever-present grain elevator punctuating the flat horizon. Visible for miles, they are beacons offering promise of hot coffee and bathrooms ahead.

Signs along Minnesota 11 announced Warroad as "Hockeytown, USA." Mainly, I presumed, because Christian Brothers manufactured hockey sticks there. Warroad boasts that adjacent Lake of the Woods has the most shoreline of any freshwater lake in the United States. This includes the shorelines of more than 14,000 islands within the lake, however. Seems like a chamber of commerce "padding" of statistics.

When I biked past Swede Carlson Field just outside Warroad and saw a few small planes on the airstrip, I thought about flying for the first time since I had flown to Wolf Point to begin this trip. At that time only one month had elapsed since I earned a pilot's license, so I had set a goal to fly at least once a month during my ride to maintain minimal proficiency.

Regulations require a pilot to fly a checkout with an instructor before renting a plane. This often takes two hours, one on the ground reviewing flight rules, airplane performance characteristics, and emergency procedures. The

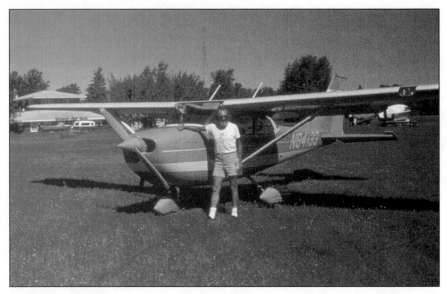

I flew a rented Cessna from Warroad, Minnesota, across Lake of the Woods to the northernmost point in the lower forty-eight states. I celebrated my first landing on a grass field. (Courtesy of Henry Kliner)

second hour involves flying a series of maneuvers and landings with the instructor. The total cost was about seventy dollars, and a flight would give me the opportunity to see and photograph the countryside. Considering this, I rented a Cessna 172 for forty dollars an hour and hired instructor Henry Kliner to accompany me for fourteen dollars an hour.

Once in the air I began reading the instrument panel aloud. Henry grinned, "I see your instructor did a good job." Then he inserted cardboard covers over all the instrument readouts. "Now, just listen to Old Betsy. She'll tell you what to do. I want you to know that you can fly without all those instruments. Flyin' is supposed to be fun."

Later, taking Henry at his word, I descended for photos of sapphire lakes, emerald islands, and sailboats. Landing on a short grassy airstrip near the community of Northwest Angle, I achieved my goal to reach the northernmost point of the lower forty-eight states. We flew over Fort Saint Charles on nearby Magnusson Island on the way back to Warroad. The fort was built in 1732 as a base for exploration and to keep peace among the Indians. In 1736 a Sioux war party massacred twenty-one Frenchmen. They were buried under the fort's chapel, "awaiting the coming of friendly hands to be gathered and given a more worthy burial place," according to Earl Chapin's book, *The Angle of Incidents: The Story of Warroad and the Northwest Angle.*

Abandoned in 1760, Fort Saint Charles was forgotten until Jesuit priests from Manitoba relocated it in 1908 after a long search. The Frenchmen's bones were dug up and moved to Saint Boniface College where they were promptly destroyed in a fire. So much for "a more worthy burial place"!

The sixty-five-minute flight cost $57.24. I was spared the stress of navigating over unfamiliar country, had someone to take the controls when I operated the camera, and received a critique of my piloting. Definitely the way to go, and the procedure I followed for the rest of my flights while biking around the United States.

Back in town, I discovered the origin of the name "Warroad." The Sioux often invaded this Chippewa territory to get to the lake's wild-rice fields. They came by way of the Red and Roseau Rivers that became known as the Old War roads.

After leaving Henry, I biked four hours before setting up camp in Beltrami Island State Forest. A nearby dining room supplied a feast of charcoal-broiled fillet of walleye, melt-in-your-mouth baked Idaho potato, a garden-fresh tossed salad, and a glass of sauvignon blanc. Before falling asleep in my tent it occurred to me I wasn't roughing it all that much. But it had been a worthwhile day: I flew more than 100 miles, collected much information, talked with interesting people, took dozens of photos, and biked forty-six miles.

歶 歶 歶

Like a short hyphen jammed sideways against State Highway 11, a gas station, hotel, bar, restaurant, and Laundromat constituted the entire business district of Williams, Minnesota.

While eating breakfast there, I visited with eighty-eight-year-old Jim Hawks, an encyclopedia of the interesting and colorful. "Glaciers made the ridges on my farm north of here," he told me. I suspected the ridges were what glaciologists call "recessional moraines." Jim described the process in picturesque fashion: "It happened like when you throw slop water out the back door in wintertime. Each time, some water freezes on top before the rest slides off the sides and leaves sort of a ridge."

I relayed this explanation to geologist friends back at the university but doubt if they incorporated it into their lectures. Today's students would find it difficult to visualize throwing slop water out the back door.

Glacial meltwater drained down and cut out the valley, Jim explained. Later, beavers built dams at frequent intervals. Each dam site created good conditions for the development of peat. Jim bulldozes the surface peat into windrows and burns it because the peat is too fine to farm. While 'dozing, he can locate each ancient beaver dam because the peat is ten- to twelve-feet deep over them, and only two to four feet elsewhere. Alert and vigorous, Jim interprets his land well.

As I prepared to leave the cafe, Peter Joslyn of El Segundo, California, rode up on his touring bike. He was forty-nine years old, broad-shouldered, handsome, and tanned, and wore sharp white shorts and a polo shirt. I felt old, short, and rumpled, as if I'd just jumped out of a dirty clothes bag.

Peter, with limited time for this adventure, had covered 4,000 miles in two months, averaging eighty to ninety miles a day. Yesterday he rode 136 miles. My record of 87.4 miles in one day seemed puny.

🚲 🚲 🚲

East of Baudette it was hot and humid. Sweat dripped from every pore. Suddenly I noticed that a carnival of colors surrounded me. Earth tones, from light tan to dark brown, bespoke the diversity of soils underlying summer-fallowed fields. A wide spectrum, from light to dark green, revealed different planting times. Newly emerged spring-planted wheat was still light colored and contrasted sharply with the darker green of fields planted last fall and beginning growth earlier this spring. Intensely yellow fields of mustard brightened the landscape. Light-green deciduous forests and dark-green coniferous forests intermingled. Red scarves of roses wrapped around fields and forests. White asters along roadsides masqueraded as satin bedspreads, stitched with purple gentians my imagination fancied as embroidered French knots.

Private enterprise flourished at a craft center in Birchdale, thanks to a group of older citizens. Needlework, woodwork, artwork, pottery, and you-name-its were offered for sale. Folks, some local, others just passing through, sat at long tables visiting and enjoying ham, eggs, and toast at reasonable prices.

A tourist discovered something she wanted. Coffee abandoned, a Birchdale entrepreneur made a sale and exchanged grandchildren stories with her customer. I watched, listened, and enjoyed a cup of coffee with a big ex-lumberjack. We talked of crosscut saws, cant hooks, and other tools of the trade once we discovered we both had worked as lumberjacks in the forests of Idaho before World War II.

A few miles before International Falls I rolled up to the Junction Tavern in Pelland in a drenching rainstorm. After peeling off wet Gortex and waterproof booties, I draped them over a bar stool and ordered a beer. An old fellow sitting at the bar said, "Kinda wet to be ridin' a bike, ain't it?" Without waiting for an answer, he continued, "Name's Joe Mannausau. M-a-n-n-a-u-s-a-u. What's yours?" That settled, Joe asked, "Where you headin'?"

"Well, from here I'll go to Maine, then down to Florida, then across to the Pacific Coast at San Diego. From there I'll head up the coast to Seattle, then pedal to Colorado, where I live."

"Did you say 'pedal'?"

"Yeah."

"Are you crazy?" Not getting a denial, Joe continued, "I thought you were on a motorcycle." A couple of guys at the bar turned with looks of disbelief.

"Why ride a bicycle?" Joe asked.

"Needed the exercise."

"Well, you'll sure get it, if you don't die of pneumonia ridin' in storms like this." Turning to the bartender, he ordered, "Hey, Ron, get this guy another beer while I take him over and buy his breakfast."

Shrugging off my protests, Joe walked me across the room to a card table where five-dollar tickets were being sold for the town's annual barbecue. What a breakfast! Barbecued beef, chicken wings, homemade potato salad, pickles, homemade rolls, and coffee.

Joe left his friends and came over to sit beside me at a long table. "How old are you?" he asked.

"Be sixty-three in a couple of weeks."

"You're old enough to have better sense. I'm eighty. I'd never try a thing like that—even twenty years ago."

Feeling Joe's energy and exuberance, and looking into his twinkling eyes, I wasn't so sure.

In *The Greening of America,* Charles Reich claims that Western society has undergone a "major change of values in which scientific technique, materialism, and the market system became ascendant over other, more humanistic values." Despite this, he concludes that some Americans still have "a consciousness which was appropriate to the nineteenth-century society of small towns, face-to-face relationships, and individual economic enterprise."

Dr. Bernie Siegel, in *Love, Medicine and Miracles,* suggests that his readers ask themselves, "Do I want to live to be a hundred?" Most, Dr. Siegel reports, will say, "Well, yes, as long as you can guarantee I'll be healthy." Most Americans, he found, were unwilling to accept all the risks and challenges of life with no such warranty. But when he asked the same question in rural areas of the world, he found that self-reliant folks, especially the older ones, looked to the future with confidence and enthusiasm.

Eighty-eight-year-old Jim Hawks in Williams, eighty-year-old Joe Mannausau at the Junction Tavern in Pelland, and the seniors in Birchdale's Craft Center reflected the conclusions of both Reich and Siegel.

A few miles down the highway, I stopped. For some reason I was numb. I couldn't feel where "things were." I recalled *Keeping the Rider on the Ride,* a humorous but useful booklet by an M.D. named Spence who was founder and president of Spenco Medical Products. This firm manufactured my padded seat cover, handlebar grips, biking gloves, and the powder for my crotch. In his booklet, Dr. Spence described an affliction of male bicycle riders as "a feeling there is nothing down there," calling it "penile numbness."

Before recalling Dr. Spence's apt description, I had thought the numbness was due to an incident a few days earlier. I had stopped for routine roadside relief when a car broke over the hill and I quickly zipped up, vaguely noting a stinging sensation. Later, chilled to the bone, I stopped at a bar in Clyde, North Dakota, where the barmaid generously agreed to brew a pot of coffee. Feeling a strange stickiness, I visited the restroom to make an inspection. Blood soaked the front of my shorts. The zipper had cut a half-inch gash across the end of my penis. Next time, the hell with modesty. But the incident convinced me I should buy a pair of more modern biking shorts that had no zipper!

In the evening, a young helper at Arrowhead Lodge on Lake Kabetogama in Minnesota removed the panniers and started to roll my bike into a storage building. Too late I yelled, "Don't touch my bike!" It took a half hour to remove the rear wheel, disentangle a bungee cord from the chain ring, and adjust the derailleur he had fouled up as well.

Making bike repairs that night was a good occasion for reflection. I had spent two hours visiting historical sites, two hours at the Junction Tavern, stopped for photos, made new friends, and rode 97.4 miles, many in pouring rain. A grin of satisfaction masked my fatigue.

🚲 🚲 🚲

East of Tower, I recoiled at the sight of roadsides scarred by clear-cut forests. The countryside was dotted with eroded logging roads, trees cut close to the highway, scattered slash, bulldozed piles of stumps, and unsightly log landings. In the early 1940s when I felled timber for the Weyerhauser Company in Idaho, these practices were common. Today, we know better than to use such damaging procedures.

After checking into Westgate Motel in Ely, I called Elizabeth, widow of Sigurd F. Olson. We knew of each other through a mutual friend. Later, I rode out to her home for tea, cookies, and conversation. I had admired Sig's writing for many years. He wrote *The Singing Wilderness* in 1956 and several other popular books on natural resources, particularly the wilderness.

Sig served as president of both the National Parks Association and the Wilderness Society, was appointed to national advisory boards, and often testified before congressional hearings. He also helped to prod Congress into designating the Boundary Waters Canoe Area Wilderness in northern Minnesota.

On the day he died, Elizabeth told me, they had been trying out new snowshoes on the wooded hills behind their home. Elizabeth's snowshoes didn't fit so she returned to the house to adjust them. Sig continued on. When he didn't return, friends began a search and found him lying in the snow. At eighty-two he had died of a heart attack while tramping in the woods he loved so much.

Elizabeth led me from her house through a forested area to "the shack" where Sig wrote his books. A woodstove, wooden shelves laden with books, an old chair, and a heavy table with a typewriter on top dominated the one-room cabin. Elizabeth removed the dustcover from the old Royal, revealing a sheet of paper in the machine. Matter-of-factly she said, "This room is just the way it was the day Sig died. Other than family and a few close friends, you are the first to see what Sig had written just before buckling on his snowshoes. Somehow, I wanted you to read it."

One line was on the paper: "A new adventure is coming up and I know it will be a good one."

I fought for composure while thanking Elizabeth for sharing such a personal matter. Ten years earlier, my seventeen-year-old son had climbed a high mountain, alone. While sitting on the tundra, watching a sunset, and listening to the haunting sounds of coyote "music," he wrote the following words in his notepad:

> *The mountain is conquered*
> *My sky is red*
> *Peaceful giant*
> *and nothin's said.*
> *Star-gazing wanderer is what I am.*
>
> *Eternal heaven grasps my mind*
> *and carries it to a starburst field of flowers.*
> *Can't count the hours*
> *And the ebony god grants a vision.*
> *My soul is arisen.*
>
> *Flightless clouds in timeless night*
> *suspend me with them*
> *Such unearthly delight is mine.*
> *Perhaps a sign.*
> *Silver threads of a golden dream surround me.*
> *My being will be free.*

Just two weeks later a drunken driver took Mark's life.

Long after leaving Sig's writing cabin, I strongly felt the presence of both this remarkable eighty-two-year-old man and my beloved son.

Later in Ely, I visited the auditorium at the Voyageur Visitor Center to see *The Wilderness World of Sigurd F. Olson*, narrated partly by Sig. Twenty minutes later the charming visitor center guide, Nancy Salsbury, gently awakened me.

"The show is over, Mr. Smith." The cumulative effect of pedaling long days had finally caught up with me.

After the short movie, Nancy and I went through a botanical collection to identify two attractive roadside plants I'd puzzled about. They were orange hawkweed and oxeye daisy. I would appreciate them even more now that I could call them by name.

The next day was the Fourth of July so I decided to stay in Ely a second day. After dumping everything out of the panniers, I laundered dirty, sweaty clothes; bought tapes, film, and other supplies; wrote several letters and mailed them, along with completed tapes and exposed film. Afterward, I reorganized my gear and oiled and adjusted Old Faithful. I also found time to feel guilty for not grinding out a few miles that day.

CHAPTER THREE

Great Lakes Region

It is inconceivable to me that an ethical relation to land can exist without love, respect, and admiration for land, and a high regard for its value.

—Aldo Leopold,
A Sand County Almanac

The fragrance of spruce, fir, and pine surrounded me as I crossed the Kawishiwi River on Highway 1 southeast of Ely, Minnesota. I inhaled deeply. Wind murmured in the treetops. Rustling leaves in the underbrush betrayed the unseen presence of a small animal. Perhaps it was a cottontail. Scratching sounds attracted my attention in time to spot a red squirrel scrambling up a red pine. Shrill birdcalls and the throaty "ker-lunk, ker-lunk" of frog talk punctuated these gentler sounds.

Earlier I had seen a deer after hearing it crash through the brush. The musky odor of a marsh prompted me to stop and peer carefully through a thin veneer of roadside trees. Beyond the trees were colorful waterfowl and shorebirds chatting and feeding in a small pond. A seldom-seen pileated woodpecker caught my attention with its distinctive hammering—loud, slow, softer at the end.

A variety of native fruiting plants—blueberry, raspberry, Juneberry, and others—tempted me from the roadside. Yielding, I stopped to snack on a handful of juicy wild strawberries.

Showy orange hawkweed and vibrant oxeye daisies flaunted their petals, dazzling the eye. These plants arrive early in a successional process that begins on disturbed sites such as cutbanks and graded roadsides. Called "pioneers," they form a beachhead of sorts. Following these hardy pioneers are plants, mostly legumes such as clover, that extract unusable nitrogen from the air and, through bacteria residing on their roots, convert it to a usable form in the soil. This provides a natural fertilizer.

Quietly rolling around a curve, I interrupted a Cooper's hawk snacking on an eastern cottontail beside the road. The cottontail had been nibbling on a salad of wild clover before his untimely end. These tasty plants are rooted in nutrient-rich soil. I had glimpsed a small skein in an intricate web of life.

As I turned into White Pine Picnic Area, a ruffed grouse led her brood of ten chicks along the forest border. The babies darted everywhere, exploring rocks, twigs, flowers, and blades of grass. The mother attempted to keep order by clucking disapproval or administering disciplinary pecks to her exuberant youngsters. As I steadied myself for a photo, two couples pulled up in a camper and the feathered family disappeared among the trees. "Was that a ruffled grouse and her babies?" asked one of the ladies. Without correcting her terminology, I admitted that the grouse probably was "ruffled."

"Oh, I'm so sorry we spoiled your chance for a picture. I'll go in the woods and drive them back." That strategy was doomed to failure, but I didn't have the heart to tell her.

Turning my attention and camera to a grove of statuesque, ancient pines, I thought about the need to preserve areas like this. Not only are they valuable for public use and enjoyment, but they also preserve some of our country's natural heritage. Seldom, if ever, will we again see a 200-foot eastern white pine. When they reach a height of seventy feet or so, consumer demands will encourage cutting for veneer, plywood, laminated beams, and other products.

In the early 1850s Congress and the public believed pine forests in the lake states would supply the needs of a growing country forever. But unwise logging practices left a cutover wasteland by the end of the century. The U.S. Forest Service now practices "sustained-yield management," claiming it will assure healthy forests in perpetuity. Only time will tell.

Near the west shore of Lake Superior, I found Two Harbors Post Office and picked up my first mail on this trip. The postmaster said there was a message to call a number in Saint Paul. Puzzled, I dialed and a voice answered, "This is Bob Linsmayer. Two days ago my son Rob called to say that he had met a bicyclist who said he would pick up his mail in Two Harbors. Rob thought I should get to know you. Can you have dinner with my wife and me in Duluth tomorrow at nine? We can meet you at the Pickwick Restaurant. We'd like to have you spend the weekend with us at our north shore home."

Bob and his wife, Christine, met me at the Pickwick, as promised. Bob is president of Villaume Industries in Saint Paul. Christine is a descendant of the Villaume family that migrated to Saint Paul from France in 1870. Establishing the business, they first manufactured only the beer boxes used in those days, then progressed to expensive paneling and doors and finally, reinforced trusses for residential and commercial construction.

The Linsmayer home has vaulted ceilings and commands an imposing view of Lake Superior. It is in a 15,000-acre private forest shared with sixty other members of the Encampment Forest Association. Christine knew how to make a dirty cyclist feel right at home: "I imagine you would like a shower tonight and to launder some clothes in the morning. Here's the bathroom. Towels are in those cabinets. You'll find detergent and cleaning supplies on a shelf in the laundry. The coffeemaker is on the counter and coffee is underneath. Get whatever you need out of the refrigerator and cupboards. We sleep in late when we're up here."

After brewing coffee early the next morning, I hiked on forest trails crisscrossed with deer and moose tracks. Ruffed grouse exploded into whirring flight from logs beside the trail. Songbird carillons rang in a new day from the forest edges. Aspen, birch, red and white pines, spruce, balsam fir, and northern white cedar blended in a delightfully variegated tapestry of greens. I had lived a whole day before breakfast!

Returning, I cleaned the bike panniers and put two loads of sweat-soaked clothes through the washer and dryer. Meanwhile, the Linsmayers and I became acquainted over sweet rolls and coffee.

Bob's interests were eclectic. He was involved in a program that provided job training, employment, and other improvements for Native Americans. Seeing future need for energy from many sources, he recently had purchased a hydroelectric plant in North Carolina that had not produced power for twenty years. With boyish enthusiasm he described scrounging around the country to locate turbines, finally finding them in Idaho Falls, Idaho.

In the afternoon, we hiked through Encampment Forest while Bob asked for my advice about wildlife and forest management. It is said that an "expert" is anyone over a thousand miles from home, so I comfortably assumed that role.

I must admit to a long-held bias that industrialists have a weak environmental conscience and little interest in social justice. That view clearly didn't apply to Bob.

Christine and Bob drove me back to Duluth, and I resumed pedaling the next morning.

Approaching the heavily trafficked Arrowhead Bridge over the Saint Louis River, I became a bit nervous. It is long, narrow, and the road climbs steeply on the other side. Four minutes later, I had made it to Wisconsin.

Wisconsin comes from an Algonquin word that means "meeting of the waters." I stopped at a street corner in Superior and asked an old man, "Why is Wisconsin called the Badger State?"

"'Cause there are so many of the dad-blamed critters. They're everywhere."

Later I checked at a library and found that the sobriquet refers to the badgerlike diggings by Welsh miners recovering shallow deposits of lead during the mining rush of the 1820s.

I wandered back roads through Oakland, Hawthorne, and Lake Nebagamon, encountering heat, humidity, hills, and mosquitoes. At Bois Brule Campground, I pitched my tent and jumped into the river for a swim. Black clouds rolled in as I left the water. Soon the wind screamed overhead, thunder crashed, and rain pounded my tent.

۰۰   ۰۰   ۰۰

After two days and 125 miles in Wisconsin, I crossed the Montreal River into Michigan, where the many Indian tribes once living along Lake Superior have contributed to the region's rich heritage of colorful place-names. Here it was Gogebic County. This Chippewa name means "body of water hanging on high." I asked folks what *that* meant. One fellow thought that 1,722-foot Mount Zion, the highest peak in the Gogebic Range, had something to do with it.

In the village of Thomaston I found a place that served a good kielbasa, a Polish sausage. The bartender was in her late twenties. Her eight-year-old son whined, "Mama, gimme a quarter to play pool."

"Don't bother me. Can't you see I've got a customer?"

She took my order and served me promptly, but her dull blue eyes seemed like windows to an empty room. Seated arms-length from a small television set, she flipped channels, never looking at her son or me, only at the flickering screen. The boy kept asking for money. His mother kept ignoring him.

Finally I blurted, "Your son has an important question to ask."

Without taking her eyes off the TV or telling me to mind my own business, she asked him, "What d'ya want?"

"A quarter, Mama."

She fumbled in her pocket and handed him a coin. He disappeared toward the back of the bar.

Some emotion prompted her to turn abruptly and state flatly, "Y'know, I lived down the road a ways ever since I was born." With that she turned silently to the screen.

Down the road "a ways" later, I pondered this vignette of life. I had thought about telling her of my two sons with whom I'd done much but now wish it had been more. But I decided not to share such personal feelings.

Later I wondered if I should have spoken up. Would the example of my sons have made a difference to a young life and a lonely lady? I'll never know.

🚲 🚲 🚲

At Presque Isle Campground, I set up camp and dined on beef jerky, trail mix, a granola bar, two Grandma's cookies, an apple, and an orange. Finished, I turned my attention to the scene around me. Couples were building campfires, cooking, riding bicycles, and walking hand-in-hand around the campground.

Grabbing my camera, I walked to the mouth of Presque Isle River to photograph the glowing sunset, then sat in thought until tinted reflections on Lake Superior blended into darkness. Filled with memories, I walked slowly back to camp where Tom and Pat Waltz from Grand Rapids invited me to their camp for a beer. Another couple dropped by and told of meeting a bear on the trail, thus starting a succession of bear stories, each more dramatic than the one before. The stories, the beer, and the camaraderie around the flickering campfire were therapeutic. I slid into my sleeping bag, feeling better.

The next morning, torrential rain greeted me. Protected by rain gear, I crossed Little Iron River, Big Iron River, Mineral River, Pine Creek, Duck Creek,

Halfway Creek, Town Line Creek, Little Cranberry River, Big Cranberry River, Floodwater River, Potato River, Weigel's Creek, Dreiss Creek, and Ontonagon River—all in the first fourteen miles. At least the rain had places to go!

◶ ◶ ◶

At breakfast in Ontonagan, two men at a nearby table described the region's economy. White Pine Copper Company, they told me, once employed 3,000 workers. Now only 300 worked there because of dwindling markets for copper. Making matters worse was the recent failure of the miners' union to renegotiate a contract. Half the local employees were on strike.

The Champion Paper Mill, which I passed on the way into town, was the major employer, but declining sales of wood products had caused a workforce reduction there, too.

Weakening markets for iron, copper, and wood products meant fewer shipments, so the Upper Peninsula Shipping Company closed down, adding to the local depression. Estimates of unemployment ranged from 20 to 30 percent.

Vicky Perron, owner of the Ontonagon Motel where I stayed overnight, wasn't sympathetic. "Workers went on strike for higher wages two years ago though they were getting about fourteen dollars an hour. Many locals were happy to get half that for steady work."

"What happened when they went on strike?" I asked.

"The union paid subsistence salaries for a year. Then the strikers got six months of welfare. That ended and there was gloom everywhere. You can blame the union. It always wants more. More money, more vacations, and more benefits."

Whatever the causes, many people were out of work in Ontonagon.

◶ ◶ ◶

Steady rain had stopped work and lumberjacks packed Jake's Bar on State Highway 26 near Winona, Michigan. I was barely inside the door when a burly fellow they called Big John turned slowly on his bar stool and growled, "How'n hell do they know where to send your Social Security checks?" There went my ego that had grown each time I heard, "Can't believe you're that old!" Big John was either a better judge of age than most, or more candid.

I ordered a beer. It arrived with three more paid for by men along the bar. I protested, "Only one. I'm driving today."

"Gotta get back in the saddle again," I announced later when the rain finally quit.

"Have a safe trip."

"Watch these rough roads and those damn trucks."

"Be careful, y'hear?"

ڿ ڿ ڿ

Slanting northeast through Upper Michigan's Keweenaw Peninsula, I rode down State Highway 26 toward Lake Superior. Bright red strawberries nestled in green-leaved clusters within inches of the blacktop. Stopping to savor their wild sweetness, I felt sorry for travelers imprisoned by automotive glass and steel. Cedar, spruce, oak, birch, and maple trees were so close to the highway that branches often brushed my helmet or leg. With this stunning beauty surrounding me, I remembered times when Carol and I had shared a similar enjoyment of the natural world.

Deep in thought, I sped around a rocky point overlooking the lake and failed to brake. Tears from the wind in my eyes and emotions in my heart streamed down my cheeks. Suddenly, as I nearly lost control, a seductive notion grasped me. Why not just let the bike crash into the rocks far below and end this damn loneliness?

I swerved toward the embankment, and tires bit into gravel. As instinct for self-preservation overcame emotion, I fought the front wheel savagely, slithering close to the brink. I lurched back to the blacktop, then into the next pull-out. Shaken, breathing hard, I realized this fleeting thought was not my way of handling problems. I gazed down at Agate Harbor with its tiny rock and pine-covered islands. The fog-shrouded vista was surreal and lovely. I could hear the lake breathing softly in the distance and its waves crashing against the cliffs below. Lake Superior was alive. And so was I!

ڿ ڿ ڿ

I arrived at Copper Harbor near the tip of Keweenaw Peninsula midafternoon. This tourist mecca sprang into being when copper ore was discovered in 1843. It peaked as a lusty boomtown five years later. Today, the saloons, livery stables, and whorehouses are gone.

At nearby Lake Fanny Hooe Campground, I pitched my tent and crawled inside just as wind and rain began slamming it. Later, I sloshed through the rain to the Laundromat, a dry place to catch up on letter writing while two loads of clothing churned through the machines.

After the rain stopped, I rode along the main drag of Copper Harbor looking for a restaurant. A van stopped beside me. It was Pat and Tom Waltz, who had invited me to their campfire for a beer and conversation on that lonely evening at Presque Isle Campground three days before. Pat said, "When we woke up, you had gone and it was raining. Tom was worried, so he drove miles hoping to find you so he could put your bike in the van and take you wherever you were going. Now we'll at least get to take you out to dinner." Their treat of whitefish orange almandine was surpassed only by quality of the conversation.

Back in my tent a lessening wind and gently falling rain lulled me to sleep. I dreamily gave thanks for the extraordinary kindness of so many strangers on this trip. The heaviness in my heart lifted and I felt enthused about continuing on.

After a fifteen-mile ride the next morning and with a healthy appetite, I parked in front of Shoreline Cafe in Eagle Harbor. After wolfing down greasy bacon, greasy hash browns, greasy eggs, and heavily buttered toast sitting in grease, it was hours before I felt healthy again. Shoreline Cafe got a four-raspberry rating.

Fitzgerald's, later in Eagle River, was better. I had strawberry pie a la mode, coffee, and conversation with Kim, the personable waitress. Owner Jim Lomat came to my table and shared his skiing adventures in Winter Park, Colorado. A four-star rating for Fitzgerald's.

By early afternoon I was hungry again. Old Country Haus Restaurant in Allouez looked inviting. When bicyclists Gene and Patty Lawershell rode up, they saw my heavily loaded bike and came in looking for me. I enjoyed *Kassler rippchen* (smoked pork ribs), as Gene told me that he teaches economics and U.S. government at Calumet High School. He is training for a triathlon. He urged me to ride back to the lakeshore and stay at McLain State Park. "It's far-ther but the ride is spectacular," Gene promised.

It was dark when I pitched my tent at McLain. Neighboring campers asked if I'd had supper and came to my rescue with a warm pasty—meat pie—they insisted was extra. It had been a day of gastronomic excess, but I slept soundly while high winds and heavy rain buffeted my tent.

Rain continued the next morning as I rode into Houghton to complete the Keweenaw circuit. Seeking a dry haven, I squished into Houghton Library, where a delightful librarian hung up my soggy outer clothing and found a dry place in the library for the bike. I wrote a few letters, then asked if they had my book *Above Timberline: A Wildlife Biologist's Rocky Mountain Journal,* which chronicled the five months I had spent alone in an old log cabin in Colorado while filming for a television documentary. To my surprise they had two copies, both checked out.

The rain finally stopped and I headed southeast on U.S. 41. Soon it was pouring again, so I stopped at the Chippewa Motel in Chassel. Having ridden and camped in the rain for several days, I decided to dry out and sleep in a bed for a change. Owner Helen Barkkari assessed my bedraggled appearance and suggested I throw my wet clothing and gear into their dryer.

"They're too dirty," I protested.

"Well, toss 'em in the washer and then use the dryer."

Later, Helen saw me putting white and colored clothing into the washer together and announced firmly, "You've just met a woman who won't let you mess up your laundry." She hauled my clothes out, separated them, and said, "You look beat. Go take a shower and a nap. I'll let you know when your clothes are finished."

A few hours later I heard a tap on my door. Helen had my clothes, all clean, dry, and neatly folded. It was great to be a "kept" man, if only while sleeping alone in a motel on a rainy afternoon.

Before turning south toward Lake Michigan, I visited Cusino Wildlife Research Station, where biologist Lou Verme described a grouse habitat proj-ect near the George E. Bauer Seney Stretch Roadside Park. He suggested I look for sharp-tailed grouse north of the road. Arriving at the park, I leaned my bike against a picnic table and asked a young couple eating lunch, "Would you watch my bike for a few minutes?"

"Sure, glad to."

I headed north on foot through a humid countryside covered with weeds and brush. The sandy soil was speckled with charcoal, the evidence of past wildfires. Thistles and raspberry bushes scratched my legs as I flushed two sharptails and found a dusting site, but it took longer to find my way back than intended. No one was at the table where my bike still leaned. A woman sitting at a nearby table called, "The young couple at your table had to leave, so we volunteered to watch your bike until you got back. Did you find any grouse?"

Seney National Wildlife Refuge provided an opportunity to stretch my legs on a short nature trail encircling a wildlife-rich pond. For an hour I sat on a log as the lowering sun splashed its golden rays across the water. Mallards and black ducks noisily cruised the marshy margins. They, too, were seeking a place to spend the night.

It was late when I reached Milwaugele Campground near Germfask, named from the first letters of the surnames of eight early settlers. A man and his two teenaged sons saw me setting up camp in the dark. They came over to visit and told me they were on a bike trip to Canada. At daybreak I watched as father and sons powered their heavily loaded bikes up the rocky path out of the campground. A year ago that sight would have been a painful reminder of losing my own two sons. Now I smiled with admiration at their good father-son relationships and remembered.

After riding eighteen miles, I was ready for breakfast in Knotty Pine Restaurant at the junction of State Highway 149 and U.S. 2. With eager anticipation, I leaned the bike in front of a window where I could watch it from inside. The enticing smell of bacon and eggs greeted me. A man, whom I took to be the owner, cook, and waiter, also greeted me. "Take that damn bike away from the front of my building," he growled.

Taken aback, I mumbled, "Had trouble with bicyclists?"

"Don't matter. I paid 7,000 dollars to paint this building. I don't want your damn bike scratching it up. You're welcome, but move that bike."

Breakfast, I decided, could wait. I pulled on my gloves, walked out, and rode on without a word. My temper has flared over less, but this was different. I'd been riding with memories of my honeymoon near here forty years ago. After those tender feelings so near the surface, I simply couldn't face a hassle. Had the man been courteous, I would have explained that only a sleeping bag and foam pad touched his building.

Al Schievenin was having coffee when I pulled into Garden Corners for breakfast an hour later. Al, owner of the nearby White Birch Resort, offered an explanation for the unfriendly treatment. "The owner of Knotty Pine is a dour character," Al said. "But we get lots of cyclists riding U.S. 2, and local business people are fed up with them."

A sharp retort was on the tip of my tongue when Al continued, "Some pull up, lean their bikes against walls, fences, trees, whatever. They come in, tie up the restrooms, leave them filthy, then ask you to fill their water bottles. Often they leave without buying a thing." I admitted he had a point and that slobs of any sort often spoil it for the rest of us.

次 次 次

In Escanaba, Carol's widowed sisters, Pauline and Julie, pampered me for five days. It was a good rest and an opportunity to spend time with Carol's family. On Saturday, my sixty-third birthday, in-laws from miles around came to Escanaba City Park for a picnic. Great home cooking! A huge cake decorated with a man on a bicycle and the words "Happy Birthday, Dwight" was a pleasant surprise.

All was not idyllic in Escanaba though. When I first rode into town, a carload of teenagers passed me. "Get that fuckin' bike off the street!" one screamed. Later, while returning from shopping downtown, I waited for the light at Ludington and Eighth Street, then started a left turn. Someone shouted from a car, "You dumb bastard, get the hell off the street!"

That did it! I dropped the bicycle in mid-intersection and bellowed, "Who the hell said that?"

One fellow looked guilty. I started for his door, but he gazed straight ahead and roared through the intersection, tires screeching. After the light changed, cars started coming from the other direction and I realized Old Faithful was in the middle of traffic. After retrieving her, I was yelled at by another motorist while pushing her to a service station where an attendant had seen and heard everything.

"Did you see who yelled at me?" I asked.

"Nope. But you're lucky you weren't run over."

Back at Pauline's house, still fuming, I called police headquarters to report the incident and ask what was considered the appropriate procedure for getting through that intersection. In chilly but polite terms, the officer made it clear he didn't appreciate an out-of-state bicyclist causing trouble. I persisted. Finally he said, "Well, I guess the way you did it was okay. But I have to tell you, people around here don't like cyclists, so you need to watch out for them."

"Well, I have to tell you I don't like motorists around here, so they need to watch out for me!" After this stupid comment, our conversation went steadily downhill.

Before leaving Escanaba it was good to attend mass at Saint Anne's Church with Pauline and Julie. I prayed for less anger and more patience.

Menominee was my last town in the Upper Peninsula of Michigan. Soon after I entered town on State Highway 41, some young fellows in a car yelled stridently and the driver hit the horn. "Here we go again," I thought.

There were no signs directing bicyclists off the street, but apparently they expected me to ride on sidewalks. I saw a ramp leading onto the sidewalk and took it. After a mile of bicycle ramps leading across side streets, I was riding into the setting sun. Too late, I saw there was no ramp at the next intersection and sailed off the foot-high curb with a testicle-crunching slam. The bike route had ended as it began—with no sign.

So I was in the street again. Within minutes some kids in a car yelled, "You dumb shit! Get that thing off the street."

Furious, I started looking for a phone. At Elias's Big Boy Restaurant, I called the Menominee police.

"Yes, we get complaints from bikers touring through Menominee. You're probably right that the bike route has ended out there. Yes, people here are a bit impatient. Don't let them bother you. Just stay far right and ride on the street. You're perfectly legal."

"I've had it with these punks," I said, my internal temperature rising again. "There's going to be trouble if I'm hassled one more time." Another stupid threat.

A long silence. Then, "Just stay where you are. I'll be out in a few minutes."

A squad car pulled in. "Now, what exactly do you want?" asked the cop.

"I want to ride peacefully to River Park Campground."

We developed a strategy. I rode ahead while he watched. Then he would pass, park, and watch for trouble in his rearview mirror. By the time we had hopscotched through town, I had calmed down and felt a bit foolish.

The policeman explained to the campground attendant that I needed a quiet place to camp. "We don't allow camping in the picnic area," said the attendant, "but if you say he's okay, he can stay there. It should be quiet."

As I started unloading the bike, someone yelled, "Hey, you over there!"

A man with a ponderous belly waddled toward me. I ignored him.

"Hey there," he called again.

"What in hell are you yelling about?"

"We had a fishing contest yesterday, and the fishermen cleaned their catch on the other side of those bushes. At night the wind blows off the lake, and it's going to stink like hell where you are."

Damn. I'd lost my temper again! "Thank you, sir. I sure appreciate your warning."

I hoped tomorrow would be a better day.

🚲 🚲 🚲

The next morning I pedaled south, entering Wisconsin again. A white-tailed deer bounded across the road. Another deer ignored me, then pranced gracefully into a stand of aspen. Twelve-foot swaths of mowed grass along the highway gave a manicured appearance. A light breeze kept me cool. A man called out, "Hi! How's the pedalin' this morning?"

Fields of tall corn and high-producing alfalfa, weed-free pastures, and patches of oak and aspen abounded. Well-kept homes and freshly painted barns were surrounded by flowers and shrubbery. I stopped and counted thirty silos around me. Signs over driveways trumpeted pride of ownership. "Deerings Dairy Farm—Jerry, Donna, Mike, Jim, and Ken." American flags waved everywhere. I hadn't seen such examples of pride and patriotism since leaving the prairie farms of North Dakota.

🚲 🚲 🚲

Near Taycheedah, I "honked" (cyclist language for standing on the pedals) my heavy bike up a steep hill to Nazareth Heights Infirmary to visit Sister Mary Constance, who was expecting me.

Carol and I had met Mary Constance fifteen years ago in Fort Collins after a devastating auto accident had nearly killed her. As Eucharistic ministers, we brought communion to her in the hospital for several weeks. Now she waved encouragement from the infirmary balcony.

Mary Constance reached up from her wheelchair to hug me tightly. "Breakfast is ready," she said. "Come and eat." During a simple breakfast, a sister introduced me to 125 nuns who applauded my presence. Many were in wheelchairs. More than twenty-five, Sister told me, were over ninety years old. Two had passed the century mark.

After breakfast I asked, "How have you been, Mary Constance?"

"Not bad, everything considered," she replied. Besides the crippling accident, Sister Mary Constance has multiple sclerosis and other diseases. She has endured so much and continued to suffer pain and serious illness. Yet, at age sixty-five, her tremendous spirit and sense of humor remained intact.

Humbled, I realized this fragile nun had more real strength than I.

"Mary Constance, how do you explain the joy and contentment I sense here?" I asked.

"I think it's because we love each other," she replied. "Younger or stronger nuns give the older ones an abundance of tender loving care, washing and brushing their hair, massaging aching feet, legs, hands, arms, and backs."

"What do the older and infirm nuns do?"

"When able, they help themselves and others. They do handwork for our craft shop. They pray for us. By being good and loving women, they strongly affect our entire community."

Mary Constance insisted on conducting a complete tour of the infirmary, from laundry to chapel. In the chapel, with Sister's wheelchair beside me and her thin hand in mine, I knelt and prayed in gratitude for the lives of Carol, Alan, and Mark, and for so many others who had blessed my life. Then I drifted from prayer to reflection.

From the moment I had entered the Upper Peninsula of Michigan where Carol grew up, wistful recollections of her often welled up inside me. There were tender memories of our honeymoon here in 1944. Some nights I dreamt about her.

On the other hand, an angry encounter with a driver at an intersection in Escanaba had unsettled me and a series of incidents in Menominee the night before I left the U.P. again triggered my temper.

Now in the quiet chapel with Sister Mary Constance, I silently asked forgiveness for my anger and for losing sight of the purpose for this journey.

🚲 🚲 🚲

Twenty-five miles north of Milwaukee, I was standing astraddle the bike while puzzling over my map. A leather-jacketed rider rumbled his Harley across the highway from a side road. He stopped inches ahead of my front tire. Thoughts of what I'd heard about these Hell's Angels types flashed through my mind and I looked for a rock. I'd go down fighting.

The Harley rider pulled off his helmet, smiled, and said, "Good morning." Pat Kennedy, a forty-four-year-old stockbroker, lived near the intersection and was riding to his office in Cedarburg. "I wondered if you planned to ride down this road. It has narrow shoulders and heavy traffic. My wife and I are cyclists, too. We have found that if you go east two more miles, then turn south you will have a safer, more pleasant ride." Pat's friendly suggestions caused me to rethink my prejudices against the biker crowd.

🚲 🚲 🚲

Milwaukee was my first experience of riding in a big city, and I was a bit anxious. A brochure describes it as "a blue-collar town where culture is experienced by screaming for their beloved Brewers and Bucks, either at the games or in one of its 1,650 taverns."

The city's south side is a simmering, shifting, ethnic melting pot. The black and Hispanic populations are increasing rapidly. A south side Catholic priest recently was quoted as saying, "My funerals are all Polish. My weddings and baptisms are all Hispanics."

Fortified by coffee and a sweet roll from Dunkin' Donuts, I pedaled toward my Polish sister-in-law's house on the south side. I worked my way to Seventeenth Street and arrived at Marie's, where I would stay for a couple of days. Marie, Carol's widowed sister, has lived on the south side since her wedding in 1937.

Amazingly, despite my apprehension, no motorists crowded me, no "hoods" hassled me. A fellow in a street crew even called out, "Hey, that's a great lookin' outfit. Don't git caught speedin'."

Before starting my ride, I had written to Robert Ruff, head of the Wildlife Department at the University of Wisconsin. His response to my inquiry about biking through Wisconsin was so prompt and his offer to take me fishing so warm it surprised me. Soon he would surprise me again.

The next morning, Bob brought his boat from Madison, picked up Marie and me, and drove us to Lake Michigan. Marie is not into fishing but was enthusiastic company. Twenty minutes after launching, we had a ten-pound king salmon aboard. Not big, but respectable. "This one's for you, Dwight," Bob said.

The water seemed to have more boats than salmon. "Squabbles over fishing spots and boat maneuvers have become so marked with anger, profanity, and obscenities," Bob said, "my wife no longer goes fishing with me." When both fishing and boaters had quieted down, Bob said, "You don't remember me, do you?"

"Well, I remember meeting you at a national wildlife meeting a few years ago," I answered.

"No, I'm thinking of an instance nineteen years ago. Because of the circumstances, I'm sure you don't remember. I was a student assistant in Yellowstone Park that summer. You were having coffee with Frank Craighead to discuss his grizzly bear studies when the phone rang. It was an officer in the Wyoming State Patrol. He told you that your son had been killed in an auto accident that morning.

"Your wife and other children were asleep in a tent a few miles away. Dr. Craighead and I drove out to be of help if needed when you awakened your family. We watched as you told them of the tragedy and packed up camp. Feeling your pain, I turned to Dr. Craighead and said, 'Someday I'll do something for that man.' Today was my first chance."

۞ ۞ ۞

A couple of days later I rode onto the Badger, a ferry that sails from Milwaukee to Ludington in lower Michigan. A clerk at a convenience store in Ludington advised me to stay on State Highway 10. "Other roads are graveled," he warned. "Traffic won't be heavy once you get to Scottville, but I'll tell you one thing. There's a twenty-mile stretch from Baldwin to Reed City that's mostly blacks. A lot of them young blacks is resentful and may run you off the road. Just watch yourself!" With that warning, I left Ludington, Michigan.

The black folks didn't bother me. But heat, humidity, and haze during the next three days gave me the feeling of pedaling in an endless tub of lukewarm water. Drivers kept their lights and windshield wipers on as they struggled to see through the muggy air. I attached a beacon to a rear pannier. The light blinks sixty times a minute and is visible for over a mile, according to the instructions. I hoped they were right.

Ten miles west of Baldwin on U.S. 10, I noticed a gradual decline in the quality of homes. Yards were unkempt, fields filled with weeds, and roadsides strewn with trash. People sat on front porches but none waved or called out. I felt uneasy.

A few miles down the road in Idlewild, rundown and abandoned houses lined both sides of the highway. Mangy dogs yipped at my pedals.

After turning south on U.S. 131, I rode by a dairy farm north of Barryton. The barns were sagging and unpainted, the weedy lawns unmowed.

I thought back to the prairies of North Dakota and the productive fields, tidy farm buildings, and pride of ownership among those farmers. A few days ago there were similar scenes in small towns and on farms in Wisconsin. I looked to the land for an explanation. Soils supporting the prosperous farmers in North Dakota and proud dairymen in Wisconsin were deep and rich. In this part of Michigan, soils were thin, sandy, and often infertile.

ڴ ڴ ڴ

Elisabeth Zorb was on my list of people to visit in East Lansing. I hadn't seen her since 1949 when her late husband, Gordon, and I were classmates at the University of Idaho. But Carol had kept in touch, and I knew Elisabeth was an enthusiastic cyclist. A few weeks earlier I had written to her for bike route maps of Lower Michigan. I arrived at her home in East Lansing in late afternoon and sat on the front porch until she arrived from her job as executive secretary for the president of the Coca-Cola regional office in Lansing.

We visited about the old days that evening. Next morning we biked to Rose Lake Wildlife Research Center where Gordon had conducted research for twenty years. After riding alone for 2,200 miles, it was good to ride with Elisabeth as she pointed out local scenery and lore. We noted the treelike sumac that speckled the roadsides with red and orange hues in the fall, and the light-green larch, a conifer with needles that turn yellow and drop off in winter.

Elisabeth taught me how to ride the rolling terrain more efficiently. When starting downhill, instead of resting, she advised, be willing to expend more

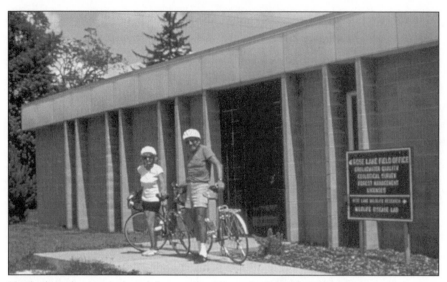

Elisabeth Zorb joined me in biking to the Rose Lake Wildlife Research Center near East Lansing, Michigan.

energy to spin in the highest gear until unable to keep up with the pedals. Then, she said, ride "low" to reduce wind resistance and coast until you can pick up the cadence and begin slamming the pedals again.

After mass on Sunday morning, Elisabeth and I visited Beal-Garfield Botanic Garden, founded in 1873. Its 5,000 plant species dazzled the eye.

I left East Lansing the next morning with a new biking technique and unexpected feelings about Elisabeth. While at the university, I had never paid particular attention to her. Now I noticed that at fifty-nine, she was still pretty, petite, and bubbling with enthusiasm. She warmly related how Carol had helped her learn to shop and told how they attended church together after she had come to this new country in 1948 to marry Gordon. They had met while he was a soldier in Germany, her native land. Passionate about bicycle touring, she asked me to stay in touch during the remainder of my journey.

Two days later I intersected the Iowa to Maine Bicycle Route at Scotch Ridge, Ohio. For the first time I used a map produced by Bikecentennial, an organization in Missoula, Montana, which later became Adventure Cycling Association.

The route followed narrow, quiet, mostly smooth roads through a countryside of farm homes, silos, and fields of corn, potatoes, and soybeans. Vast fields of cucumbers were being harvested by migrant workers from Mexico.

Using the hill-riding technique learned from Elisabeth, I developed an efficient synchrony riding the rolling hills. I would hit over thirty miles per hour at the bottom, turn on the calorie-power, and top the next hill at fifteen. Crickets sang like crazy, and a light breeze pushed from behind. Hallelujah!

🚲 🚲 🚲

A *Washington Post* reporter once described Cleveland as "this grim industrial city, a cheerless vista of abandoned factories, shuttered shops, decaying neighborhoods." I read in *The Book of America,* however, that "an emerald necklace of fine parks ... circles the city." As an ecologist I knew that beauty and biological diversity are often greatest at the edges of fields, forests, and ponds. I wondered if the concept applied to cities, too. It did—in this case, at least. Metroparks Valley Parkway was a curving, rolling, tree-shadowed bypass around Cleveland.

Leaving the bypass, I found myself in front of 72 Harriman Street in Bedford, puzzling over my map. A car turned into the driveway and the driver rolled down his window. "May I help you?" he asked.

"I'm looking for the Cee-Ray Motel. Have a reservation there."

"It's up this street a few blocks." I explained a little about my trip, and then he asked, "What time do you eat breakfast?"

"I usually ride for an hour or so, then eat about seven."

"Well, I have a prescription for you. Get some extra sleep and come back at 7:30 A.M. for breakfast. You're in front of my house."

That is how I met Marty Ruddock, a physician at a Bedford clinic. After breakfast next morning, Dr. Ruddock described his hobbies. In three typewriters were pages from three manuscripts. One title was "The Influence of Gristmills on the Development of Central Ohio." The second paper reported on "The Characteristics of Women Suffering from Bulimia and Anorexia." The third dealt with horology, which, Marty explained, was the art or science of making precision timepieces. A dozen handsome grandfather clocks stood in the den and elsewhere in Marty's home.

I was ready to leave when he offered, "I do lots of biking and know the best way to get out of city traffic. I'd like to ride with you for a few miles."

Fifteen days later I received a letter from Marty. It read, in part: "I never intended to ride thirty-one miles with you when we started, but it was such a fine day and the miles seemed to float by beneath us. You have done a great deal with your life and you continue to grow. You are older and growing as opposed to many senior citizens who are simply old and growing older."

I warmed to his praise and vowed to work harder to deserve it.

❀ ❀ ❀

Exactly forty years ago Carol and I had pledged to love each other "until death do us part." Now, August 21, 1984, I stopped at the Swiss Haus Restaurant in Geneva for dinner and a margarita, our traditional anniversary drink. Later I slept restlessly in a KOA campground, dreaming off and on of our years together.

Memories of Carol were still with me when I visited Alliance College in Cambridge Springs, Pennsylvania, two days later. The Polish National Alliance created this private school in 1912.

"This library houses one of the largest Polish studies collections in the United States," boasted the librarian. "Ignace Paderewski gave the first commencement address in 1916. Zbigniew Brzezinski, Edmund Muskie, and Lech Walesa all received honorary doctorates from Alliance."

I went to a large wall map of Poland and found Czekaj, the small town near Warsaw where Carol was born. I'd not looked it up before. Carol came to the United States with her parents when she was only a year old so didn't remember her life in Poland.

❀ ❀ ❀

After a cold but restful night in Penn Highlands Campground, I warmed up by pedaling briskly out of the valley. Brilliant sunlight and the frenzied singing of chickadees greeted me as I emerged from the clinging fog into a crisp new day. It didn't stay crisp for long. As the hills became steeper and the sun rose higher, sweat streamed down my cheeks, arms, back, and chest. Off came my warm sweats, on went a headband to keep the sweat out of my eyes. Wristbands were added to keep the sweat from running into my leather-faced biking gloves.

I hadn't realized that northwest Pennsylvania was so mountainous. Aspen, maple, pine, and hemlock covered the hills. Willows bordered sparkling streams that sliced between one steep hill after another. In this area, along Lake Erie's southern shore, edges of Ohio, Pennsylvania, and New York converge.

In Russell, it was time to pick up emergency supplies of individually packaged apple and peach pies, cheese, crackers, and fruit juices at an old-time country store. I followed the Allegheny Reservoir Scenic Drive north a few miles before reading the sign, "Welcome to New York, Mario M. Cuomo, Governor." The roaring sound of a stream cascading down the narrow valley near the road told me steeper hills lay ahead.

My mind's eye compared these hills and those for the last fifty miles in Pennsylvania with the foothills of the Rockies west of Denver. Both display a mixture of hardwoods and conifers and a sprinkling of homes, but similarities ended there. Here the homes were older, less expensive, less obtrusive. Surrounded by unpainted barns, small fields of corn and native hay, and small herds of Holsteins, Jerseys, Guernseys, and Herefords, these folks still made their living from the land. In the Colorado Rockies, affluent people buy "space" to distance themselves from others and enjoy the spectacular scenery, but they make their living elsewhere—and pollute the air commuting to work.

🚲   🚲   🚲

On a Sunday afternoon two days after entering New York state, I walked into the Turfside Restaurant near the 18th hole of a golf course. Sweat dripped on the floor as I pulled off helmet and biking gloves and sat at a table with white linen tablecloth and napkins. Moments later, a well-dressed gentleman about my age came over and invited me to join him and his wife for dinner.

Arnold Cook was chairman of the Business Administration Department at Houghton College, a Wesleyan institution twelve miles from the Turfside. His wife, Betty, taught biology, botany, and ecology there.

"We don't have any plans for this afternoon," Arnold said as we finished dinner. "I'll draw you a map to our house. When you get there, Betty and I will take you for a tour of the area."

When I strained up to their hilltop home, the Cooks were ready to go. We drove to Letchworth Park, which showcases Genesee Gorge, sometimes called the Grand Canyon of the East. In the Seneca dialect *Genesee* means "great and beautiful river." One of the three falls in the canyon cascades 110 feet and is 250 feet wide.

Next, Arnold drove to Moss Lake Sanctuary where Betty had studied bog ecology for her master's degree in biology. At a picnic table, Betty set out candles and supper while Arnold described the marsh life as we enjoyed a spectacular sunset. Then Arnold blessed the food that graced the picnic table and that filled the night air with an incense of promised flavor. The flickering candlelight reflected off the shadowing pines. As the iridescent sky slowly changed to indigo over Moss Lake, we talked softly, transfixed, filled with more than food.

The Cooks' extraordinary hospitality led to a friendship that has continued since.

ᵭᵭ ᵭᵭ ᵭᵭ

The main drag in Short Tract, New York, was empty except for a lone Holstein heifer that refused to budge as I biked around her into town. When I stopped to check my map, seventy-seven-year-old Clifford Prentice came out of his general store to visit. Clifford was born a few miles west of this village of a hundred people. Soon afterward his family moved to Birdsall, six miles east of town. In his entire lifetime, Clifford had left southwest New York state only twice, on short trips to adjacent Pennsylvania.

Trouble seemed always to follow Clifford. At age twenty-two, he and his dog were rounding up cows in a pasture when one charged. The dog darted between Clifford's legs, and the pursuing cow gored him in the crotch and leg. He's been crippled since. Nine years after this painful incident, Clifford was thrown from a bucking horse. His broken leg never healed properly. Arthritis set in, and a hip began to deteriorate. After years of hobbling around, he began using crutches in 1977. From Clifford's ruddy complexion and remarkably muscular arms, one would never guess that he has physical problems as he continues to run the store.

Clifford asked, "Tell me, what do you think of our little mountains here?"

"Well, they're not as high as the mountains in Colorado, but some of these hills are steeper than the ones at home."

"Ya don't say? Boy, I bet those Rockies are really somethin'."

As I left Short Tract, Clifford called after me, "By jiminy, I wish I was seein' the world like you're doin'!"

🚲 🚲 🚲

It was September 1 and I'd been on the road for two and a half months. The beauty along Allegheny 15A was breathtaking. Maples acknowledged autumn with hues of red and orange. Tamaracks had turned yellow. The aspen, alder, beech, ash, and oak were prettying up as well. Eastern white pines, resisting fall fashions, remained haughtily aloof in solid green. The visual splendor ended at the Keeney Wildlife Management Area sign as if banned by state statute. Nonetheless, treasures hidden from casual travelers were there.

Rich with nutrients, ponds provide food, space, and protection for hosts of wildlife species such as sunfish and bass, mallards and coots, turtles and crayfish, beavers and muskrats, to name a few. Muddy ponds, fringed with clumps of cattails, reeds, rushes, and grasses were a delight to red-winged blackbirds and migrating warblers. A great blue heron stood in a pond, regally statuesque, waiting for lunch. Apparently convinced no food was in that spot, he began stalking across the pond in slow, measured strides. Suddenly, his head darted into the water and jerked up with a tiny frog wriggling in his bill. Lunch had been served. Dead trees, spiking upward around the ponds, furnished launching platforms from which red-shouldered hawks dive-bombed for food.

🚲 🚲 🚲

On Labor Day Sunday, I breakfasted at the Farm Restaurant in Old Forge, New York, and attended mass at Saint Bartholomew Church. Later I photographed an attractive roadside sign, "Adirondack League Club." A couple on the porch of a small house near the locked gate called, "Where are you from?"

After learning I'd taught courses in ecology and wildlife management, they asked, "Do you know Dr. Dwight Webster from Cornell?"

"Only from his fisheries research."

"Well, he's our resident scientist, and he's here this weekend. We'll call him. Maybe he'll give you a tour."

After Dwight met me at the gate, we watched members race canoes on Little Moose Lake. Others played tennis on the only wood-surfaced tennis courts used for tournaments in the United States. The club formed in 1890, Dwight told me, and catered to New York's rich and powerful. Since its beginning, the Adirondack Club has championed natural resource causes and in 1950, established a memorandum of understanding with Cornell University to conduct research.

One ongoing study examines the effects of acid rain on natural fish production in lakes and streams. Another probes the possibility of developing a triploid species of trout that will be more productive. In a third investigation, the goal was to cross domestic brook trout with a wild brook trout to produce a hardier fish called Temiscamie.

The half day I spent with Dwight brought some remorse about retirement. There is great challenge in the quest for that elusive commodity called truth. Research still excites me.

Before leaving the Adirondacks, I wanted to visit Anne LaBastille, who lived on an island in Big Moose Lake. Anne studied mule deer in Colorado and received a master's degree at Colorado State University where I assisted her with fieldwork and served on her graduate committee. In twenty years as an ecologist and natural history writer, Anne studied and fought the causes of acid rain, destruction of rain forests, and steady losses of endangered wildlife. Author of several books, including the best-selling *Woodswoman,* she is an enthusiastic and articulate spokesperson for environmental causes.

In the village of Inlet I made a dozen phone calls trying to locate Anne. Finally, a doctor at Glen's Falls hospital told me that Anne had broken her leg. He gave me her phone number in Warrensburg, where she was recuperating at the home of a friend.

"Anne, what happened?" I asked. Anne explained that she had been working alone on the island when she rolled a log over her left leg. To get help, she crawled to her boat, rowed across the lake, crawled to her pickup, and drove to the hospital. She relieved the pain by sticking her left leg out the window to elevate it and used her right foot to operate the clutch, brake, and accelerator.

"I am so sorry this happened," Anne said. "Since you wrote, I've been planning to take you out to the cabin so we could catch up on the twenty years since I left Colorado." I was disappointed to miss her, but Warrensburg seemed far away and the road ahead was calling.

CHAPTER FOUR

New England

I shall be telling this with a sigh, somewhere ages and ages hence: Two roads diverged in a wood, and I ... I took the one less traveled by, and that made all the difference.

—Robert Frost,
"The Road Not Taken"

In the last section of the Adirondacks, cattails, pond lilies, and ducks appeared in the misty dawn over Lake Durant. Picking up speed from the divide between the Saint Lawrence and Hudson Rivers, I rolled down State Highway 28 in New York toward an ethereal scene.

I'd driven this highway twice before, most recently with Carol for a few days in New Hampshire and Maine while I reviewed wildlife habitat management plans and practices for the White Mountain National Forest. Both times we traveled fast, saw little, and rushed to keep our schedule. This time I followed less traveled roads more slowly. And that made all the difference.

On a thirty-eight-mile-an-hour downhill run, I came within a few feet of a sleek white-tailed doe. Startled, she leaped high in the air, then ran alongside me. I was moving too fast, though, and she fell behind. Churning along the crystal-clear Hudson River as it flowed past pine trees and reddening maples, I felt invigorated, as if I could go on forever. Then a second, more visceral sensation of hunger took over. Pancakes with maple syrup at the Adirondack Trail Coffee Shop in Indian Lake couldn't have tasted better.

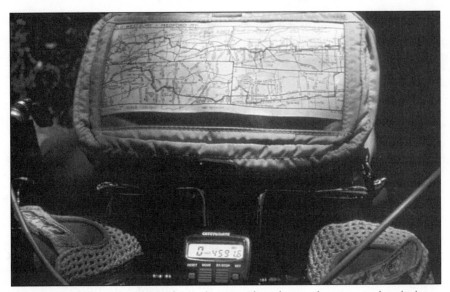

The maps for the New York part of my adventure. The odometer between my hands shows 459.18 miles.

The French used 2,000 men to construct Fort Ticonderoga in 1756 and 1757. No sooner had the ring of their hammers and axes subsided than the crack of rifle fire and thump of cannons sounded across Lake Champlain. Up until then, the region had had its share of conflict that began shortly after French explorer Samuel de Champlain discovered the lake in 1609. Champlain joined forces with the Huron and Algonquin Indians to attack the Iroquois. In the course of the battle, he killed two of their chiefs, and the Iroquois never forgot. This first experience with a white man led to the bloody French and Indian Wars.

I wandered through the fort, listening to guides and reading plaques. In its short life span, Fort Ticonderoga experienced some of the most concentrated combat of any fort in the world. Attacked six times between 1755 and 1777, the fort fell three times and held three times. At least 10,000 lives were lost in these inconclusive battles. The British were in control at the end of military action but later abandoned the fort as the French had earlier.

The next flurry of activity was in 1909 when American entrepreneurs "captured" Fort Ticonderoga. Nowadays, the occupants take aim not at enemy troops but at the tourist's wallet.

🚲 🚲 🚲

A ferry took Old Faithful and me across Lake Champlain from New York into Vermont where houses were large, square, and almost without exception, white with either gray or green roofs. Most had green or black shutters. White-spired churches, white birches, and red barns maintained the conservative scheme of things. Signs in front yards advertised beans, corn, squash, tomatoes, eggplants, cucumbers, maple syrup, and cheese for sale.

Shortly after leaving the ferry, I entered a shop looking for a midmorning caffeine fix. "We don't have any," snapped the gray-haired lady behind the counter. "I think you can get coffee at a store up the road a piece. There ain't many towns up here. You just have to plan better." While I pondered that advice, she turned to more important customers.

Bernard DeVoto, noted in the 1930s that this Vermont Yankee abruptness and character resulted from their ancestral Calvinism. He wrote, "Its philosophy that life is an endless struggle against evil and necessarily a losing one, exactly agrees with the experience of a people who settled on a thin, boulder-sown soil in a ferocious climate, where mere survival was success."

Vermonters, dismayed by the expanding interstate system and air travel that brought tourists in droves, reacted in 1970 by overwhelmingly passing Act 250, a basic land use bill. Billboard and bottle bans followed. Such progressive environmental legislation seems paradoxical for a people who cherish traditional freedoms.

Midway across Vermont, my allegiance to Colorado and the Rockies faltered. Alternate places to retire danced in my head. Middlebury's special appeal included all the amenities I'd want—skiing and hiking in surrounding mountains, a small airport nearby, world-renowned museums and art galleries, and a college noted for its language school and the prestigious Bread Loaf Writers' Conference. The quiet campus would be a fine environment for writing. Perhaps I could even teach an ecology course.

⚅ ⚅ ⚅

I met Henny from Toronto and Frank from Englewood, Colorado, who were at the Schoolhouse Hostel in Rochester, Vermont, when I arrived. We prepared our own suppers in the kitchen and compared biking notes. Henny would ride her bike to Maine for more touring. Frank, in the middle of a semester off for biking, asked her about routes to Toronto. He intended to tour Quebec with friends before returning to Connecticut College.

We discussed routes, makes of bikes, tires, gear ratios, and miles traveled. Not once did they ask my age, invariably the first question from auto and motor home tourists. It was affirming to have these young cyclists accept me for what I could do on a bicycle and not bring age into the discussion.

Still in Vermont, I struck out toward Thetford Center. After eighty days on the road, I felt supremely confident in handling eighty-five pounds of bicycle and gear. Too confident at times. Rolling downhill at forty miles an hour and finding the road rougher or a turn sharper than expected triggered huge spurts of adrenalin. Going that fast was a bit foolhardy, but it felt too good to hold back.

The feeling of having control over my body was another high. Strength and endurance had increased. I drove the pedals hard. On level terrain, with no headwind, Old Faithful rolled along at twenty miles per hour, the speed limit in some Vermont villages.

After crossing the Connecticut River into New Hampshire, I stopped in Piermont, where the bike map showed a bed and breakfast. A sign on the door read "Closed." Not to be denied, I knocked loudly. A voice behind me called, "You looking for supper and a bed?"

"Sure am."

"We have an extra bed. Come on over."

The Shields had come to my rescue. I was starting to unload when Arnold interrupted, "Looks like you could use a shower and a drink. Here, take this scotch and water into the bathroom with you. You can unpack your bike later. We'll hold supper."

While holding it, Muriel added fresh vegetables to the salad and cooked mouth-watering homemade sausage to supplement the steak intended for two. I discovered they were officers in the cycling organization League of American Wheelmen and were holding a meeting in their home that evening. Arnold commented, "We saw your camera. Do you happen to have any slides?"

"Yeah, the film processor mailed two boxes to Ticonderoga where I picked them up the other day. I haven't looked at them yet."

"Well, stick them in this carousel tray. Our meeting begins in twenty minutes and you're the program." It went over fine. An audience of enthusiastic cyclists was easier to captivate than one of my classes of 200 still-sleepy college students at eight o'clock in the morning!

The Shields's house, once a store with ballroom overhead, was later converted to apartments. The latest conversion created a long, narrow structure that looked like two homes connected by a covered breezeway. To the left of the breezeway was their home, to the right a solid door. "That leads to the only barbershop in the country with no windows," Arnold told me.

From the other side of the barbershop, another door led into the back of the post office. A former postmaster barbered surreptitiously for years without a license. He sneaked his patrons in, disguised either as guests to his home or as post office customers.

Arnold continues barbering, legally now. Sometimes local people give him a dollar or two. More often they leave a dozen eggs, a pound of homemade butter, some vegetables, or such. Over fifty years ago, my family lived like this in the mountains of Idaho. I was pleased to find this economic style still existed.

Arnold wouldn't take a penny for all the amenities of a first-class bed and breakfast, which included a huge country breakfast that Muriel prepared at 5:30 the next morning.

By midafternoon, I had approached 2,988-foot Kancamagus Pass with head down and sweat dripping. Suddenly, applause and shouts of encouragement erupted from a dozen people looking down from a turnout cut back from the summit. I pedaled up and pulled in. A burly fellow extended a cold beer and a cheeseburger just off the grill. A local motorcycle club was enjoying a cookout. My opinion of the black leather crowd inched up another notch.

ᛞᚱᛟ   ᛞᚱᛟ   ᛞᚱᛟ

In the euphoria induced by exercise and a luminous dawn, I wheeled into Fryeburg, Maine, alternately whistling at full pucker and singing at the top of my lungs. I had pedaled eighty miles, west to east across New Hampshire in one day.

Fred Westerburg came out of his store at Saco River Canoe and Kayak Landing while I photographed the huge stack of canoes out front.

"Ever see this many canoes?" he asked.

"Can't say I have."

"Where you headed?"

"Montana."

"I saw you ride in. You're headin' the wrong way for Montana."

"Well, I'm going to Maine, Florida, and California first."

"Say again?"

After I fleshed out my itinerary a bit, Fred asked one of his guides, Bob Tara, to take me on a canoe trip down the Saco River. I happily changed plans for the day.

Bob, a 275-pound defensive tackle for the Ottawa team in the professional Canadian Football League, paddled in the stern. He told me, "I pile a hundred pounds of rocks up front when canoeing with my girlfriend." I could see why. The bow tilted so high I could scarcely reach the water with my paddle.

As we paddled, Bob described several abandoned hydroelectric plants being put back into production in Maine. "When I started teaching ecology fifteen years ago," I told Bob, "there wasn't much interest in small water-powered plants. But huge hydroelectric projects were opposed by environmentalists and others who preferred free-flowing rivers. Everyone was waiting for nuclear power."

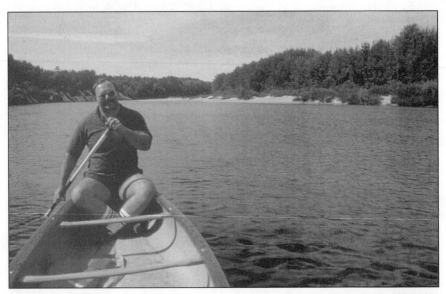

Bob Tara, a professional river guide, took me down the Saco River in Maine. Bob is also a defensive tackle in the Canadian Football League.

"Well," Bob responded, "environmental concerns and the dismal record of nuclear power plants, such as our own Maine Yankee plant, led to second thoughts by many people."

My thoughts went to my weekend in Minnesota when Bob Linsmayer told how he had bought small hydroelectric plants around the country and brought them back into production. I also thought of my conversation with doctor/author Marty Ruddock in Ohio, who spoke of his interest in old water-powered gristmills.

I wonder if we will ever suppress our expectations for high technology and go back to using clean resources such as wind and water for more of our needs? Perhaps there is some hope, but I doubt if we'll ever go back to gristmills.

🚲 🚲 🚲

Maine is a land of one-liners. At a lunch counter in Canton, I asked a huge fiftyish fellow about the route ahead. Turning the map this way and that, he kept mumbling, "This ain't right." I chuckled and told him people often went through that routine of map orientation, while I always kept north at the top when reading a map. Fixing me with a you-don't-know-much look, he growled, "Wal now, son, ya gotta know where yore ass is afore you know which way yo're pointed."

The no-shoulder road was rough between Palmyra and Newport. I was rolling down a hill, the bike jarring violently, when a truck driver hit his air horn and screamed past. All I could do was hang tough and cuss. More and more I appreciated Hartley Alley's pretrip counsel about defensive riding: "Ride far right and keep an eye on your rearview mirror if you want to stay alive on busy roads."

Rusted mufflers, broken beer bottles, stripped tire treads, orphaned hubcaps, assorted bolts, unidentified automobile innards, and an occasional dead skunk made "staying far right" more difficult than impatient motorists realized. But the joy of riding the roads outweighed these hazards.

🚲 🚲 🚲

West of Surry, small clearings hacked out of scrubby stands of black spruce, tamarack, pine, and scattered birch interrupted the forests along State Highway 178. I walked over to a man working in one of these clearings.

"Name's Gawd'n Cawdah," he introduced himself. I interpreted that to be Gordon Carter. "Ah'm fixin' mah blueberry patch," he continued.

I had no idea, though, why he was scattering hay over mowed blueberry stubble. He explained, "Ah leave it on 'til spring, then set it on fiah. That brings on the new crop."

The economics of the whole venture escaped me. This year, Gordon had harvested about 5,000 pounds of blueberries off his one-acre plot. He said berries were fifteen cents a pound. That amounts to $750 for the crop. He paid a crew $470 to pick the berries. That left $280 for mowing off the bushes, hauling hay with a pickup and trailer, spreading it with a pitchfork, and coming back to burn it next spring.

"Seems like a lot of work for the money you get out of it," I commented.

"That's awright. Ah jus' like to come up here an' spend th' day foolin' around."

Gordon had retired after thirty years with the Maine Highway Department. "Travel a lot now?" I asked.

"Nope. Drove to Washington state once."

"Ever think about going south for the winter after you're finished with the blueberries?"

"Nah. Ah got a friend who's allus runnin' around. He says Ah should travel more. But Ah got this land an' a house 'bout eight miles up the road. Y'know, ever time Ah come up, Ah see somethin' new. 'Course that's 'cause Ah'm lookin' for it."

"Looking for what?"

"Oh, new flowers, diff'rent colors, diff'rent smells, animals an' birds an' snakes an' stuff like that. Nah. Ah don't see why Ah should go runnin' around the country lookin' for new things. There's enough right here. Don't make much, but the land ain't worth much. Old folks who owned the farm died off, but the dirt already'd gone sour."

Yes, I thought, Gordon is well off here. He knows the country, knows how to see new things, and is content. Why should he "go runnin' around"?

Gordon had only one complaint, echoing what I'd heard in nearly every community: "Things are changin'. When Ah go to the store, Ah don't know nobody no more."

A half mile down the road I realized I hadn't taken a picture of Gordon so I rode back.

"Oh, that's fine if you wanna take my pitcha," he said. But I couldn't get him to pose. Instead, he busied himself with stirring the hay and only acknowledged me by laughing every time he heard the shutter snap.

After leaving Gordon, I stopped at the store in Surry for coffee, a doughnut, and a banana. Mrs. Carter was at the store. "Gordon said a bearded bicyclist took his picture."

How did she know that? Gordon hadn't passed me. He must have dropped his pitchfork once I left and gone to someone's home to call his wife. That rascal wasn't as modest as I thought!

æ   æ   æ

Kathy Dudzinski back in Fort Collins had said, "If you are near Newbury Neck, look up my dad. I'll write that you are coming."

Now I rode down Newbury Neck Road as it wound along picturesque Union River Bay. The driver of an oncoming car slammed on his brakes. It was Dr. Ben Whitcomb, Kathy's dad.

"I'm going to the post office," he said. "My wife, Peggy, will show you your room. Make yourself at home. I'll be back soon."

After visiting with Peggy, I carried all four panniers upstairs to my bedroom and arranged the contents of the fourteen compartments into fourteen piles on the floor. I reorganized each pile before packing them back into their waterproof bags. Everything in good shape, I relaxed and enjoyed the ocean view until Ben returned.

We drove to their property on the other side of the bay. It included a cottage, teahouse, boathouse, garage, and a thirty-five-foot sloop at anchor in the bay. In earlier years, Ben had raced a fifty-foot yawl with a crew recruited mostly from family members. Now he settled for sailing his sloop each year in the Old Skipper's Race along the Maine and Connecticut coast.

Ben and I drove to Ellsworth after dinner to shop. As he picked up groceries, Ben whistled, ran down the aisles with his dog, and played hide-and-seek with a delighted little girl whose worried mother obviously didn't know Ben. My spur-of-the-moment comment, "Don't worry, ma'am, your little girl won't hurt him," didn't seem to help.

Dr. Ben had trained in Hartford, Connecticut, before World War II, practiced neurosurgery at Walter Reed Hospital during the war, then returned to practice in

Hartford. Now semiretired, he drives to nearby Ellsworth to see patients one day a week. Primarily he does back surgery and a surgical technique for treating carpal tunnel syndrome, a condition that causes stiffness and swelling of hands.

"I don't practice brain surgery anymore. At seventy-six, it's time to let younger doctors have the trauma of working with serious head injury and other problems of the brain," he explained.

That evening, we looked at photos of Dr. Ben and Korczak Ziolkowski, a Polish sculptor who had died a few months before. Korczak spent his last thirty-five years carving the Crazy Horse Memorial from a 600-foot granite mountain in the Black Hills near Mount Rushmore. Many decades of work remain to complete the project.

Ben had performed three disc operations on Korczak, who later hired a professional photographer to prepare a photo album acknowledging the deep friendship binding these two talented men. To further show his appreciation, Korczak sculpted a marble bust of one of Ben's sons.

I was ready for bed when Ben appeared at the door in his pajamas. We ended the day comparing exercises to maintain strength and flexibility.

It was raining next morning when I left my bed. Ben, already in running gear, came downstairs. "Bacon and eggs are in the refrigerator," he said, "bread is by the toaster and coffee by the coffeemaker on the counter. I'll be back in a half hour." Half out the door he turned. "Peggy left early for a hairdresser appointment. She and I leave tomorrow for Germany to see the Oberammergau Passion Play." I had arrived at an inconvenient time, I realized, but Peggy and Ben never let it show.

The skies cleared at 10:00 A.M. In bright sunlight and with cool breezes blowing off Blue Hill Bay, I climbed steep hills at four miles an hour and spun down the other side at thirty-five. Continuing the Blue Hill theme, I wound through East Blue Hill, around Blue Hill Harbor to Blue Hill. Then I pedaled past Blue Hill Falls to Blue Hill Neck where State Highway 175 took me through South Blue Hill.

Sedgwick Bed and Breakfast, a charming 1826 Cape Cod home, sits on five wooded acres looking out over the Benjamin River and Eggemoggin Reach. It was a good place to spend the night.

Next morning, all I could see were cloud banks, trees bending in the wind, and heavy rains slanting earthward. Owner Kathryn Brunelle drove to town to shop and left me in a cheery guest room with a pot of hot coffee and a half-dozen cats. It should have been an ideal setting to complete the writing of a magazine article, but I was restless. Even in the rain, it was more fun to ride than to write.

Finally, the ominous clouds broke up and disappeared. Leaving a note and check for Kathryn, I pedaled on to meet Jim Gilbert. A Colorado State University graduate, Jim was now a professor at the University of Maine.

After I reached his home, Jim said he wanted to give me a close-up view of the coast of Maine from his seventeen-foot skiff. But first, he needed to go to town for new spark plugs to repair the cranky engine. Using a life preserver as a pillow, I stretched out in the bottom of the boat, intending to catch up on narrating. Instead, rocked gently by the waves and warmed by the muted September sun, I was sound asleep when Jim returned. "Hey, no sleeping on the job," he chided me.

For the rest of the day, we cruised along the rockbound coast while Jim taught me coastal ecology, a reversal of our former roles as student and teacher. Jim talked about his career as professor and researcher. Again, I felt pride in the accomplishments of a former CSU student. While listening, I photographed harbor seals and admired the quaint fishing villages we passed.

🚲   🚲   🚲

North of Orono, a truck driver hauling wood chips began hitting his horn a hundred yards behind me. In the rearview mirror, I saw him swerving toward me, then a blast of air hit as he blew past. I ended up in the ditch, flat on my back with a badly bruised ankle. "You son of a bitch," I yelled from this ignoble position. A pickup was following and the passenger called from his open window, "You tell 'im, buddy." I couldn't tell if he was sympathetic or sarcastic.

I was barely back on the road when a second truck bore down with air horn blasting. This time I kept both balance and nerve as he roared by within inches; then I spun down the road in hot pursuit, hoping to locate both trucks at a sawmill. They were nowhere to be found. Probably just as well.

My ankle was still swollen two days later when I reached East Millinocket, but I decided to keep a date with Mount Katahdin, Maine's highest peak at 5,267 feet.

I had mentioned to Jim Gilbert's wife, Donna, that one goal of my trip was to climb Katahdin. She said, "We've lived in Maine for eight years and have never gotten around to climbing it. I'll go with you."

She left home at 5:00 A.M. and drove a hundred miles to join me. We hoped for an early start but storm clouds threatened our climb. We decided to go anyway.

We enjoyed the climb up Katahdin but to emerge from the forest and walk on tundra at 5,000 feet was a new experience for me. Tundra doesn't begin until about 12,000 feet in Colorado.

Near the top, winds picked up, the temperature dropped, and clouds scudded across the summit.

Robert Frost wrote about Katahdin:

> *Oh, stormy stormy world,*
> *The days you were not whirled*
> *Around with mist and cloud,*
> *Or wrapped as in a shroud,*
> *And the sun's brilliant ball*
> *Was not in part or all*
> *Obscured from mortal view—*
> *Were days so very few ...*

Clouds also obscured our "mortal view" but cleared enough near the summit that we found a Pennsylvanian with three cameras.

"I've never climbed this high before. Would you mind taking my picture with each of these cameras?"

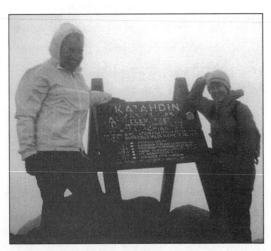

At the summit of Katahdin, Maine's tallest peak, with Donna Gilbert

I was curious why he had three cameras. But cold rain changed to chunks of sleet that whipped past our faces and splattered against the rocks, so I hurriedly clicked the shutters without asking. The Pennsylvanian took a couple of photos of Donna and me standing by the wooden marker on the peak.

My biking shoes were not designed for clinging to wet boulders and the cold sleet penetrated my light sweatpants and jacket as we started our descent. We reached Katahdin Stream Falls Campground at the base of the mountain, soaked and chilled after a slippery descent of 4,200 feet. I'd worn the seat out of my sweatpants by sliding down the face of room-size granite boulders. Donna handled the descent with more aplomb.

Pedaling eighty-seven miles the next day exceeded my expectations, but that mileage was not without cost. Sore and stiff, I toppled over twice just trying to get off my bike. My ankle felt better, though.

South along Passamaquoddy Bay, I pitched my tent at Sunset Point Park, billed as "The Easternmost Campground in the United States," then biked out to Quoddy Head State Park, where the sign read, "The Easternmost Point in the United States."

Detouring north, I crossed the graceful Franklin D. Roosevelt Memorial Bridge to Campobello Island and visited the Roosevelt "cottage," with its eighteen bedrooms.

ڪ ڪ ڪ

Three gray-haired ladies sat at a nearby table in the restaurant where I stopped for lunch. A tape recorder malfunction later obliterated my record of the name of the restaurant or the town. Considering the nature of the conversation I overheard, it is probably just as well.

The loudest entertained her companions with a story of two women who had been living in a shanty on an offshore island. "When they moved to town, they held hands ever' where. They jus' liked each other too much for folks 'round here. We saw to it there was no more of that, Ah can tell you!" As I paid my check, I wondered what the townsfolk did about it but didn't ask.

Most of the forests between Calais and Cherryfield were clear-cut decades ago, farmed awhile, then abandoned. These old fields, invaded by crimson fireweed, blue lupine, and white daisies, were pleasing to the eye, but not good for making a living. A scattering of old houses and shabby trailer homes confirmed my opinion.

In newer fields carved out of the scrubby forests of second-growth white fir, black spruce, alder, and tamarack, I saw two mowing machines and a dump rake, each pulled by a team of horses. For the next hour of pedaling, I reminisced about the 1930s, when I'd driven a team of horses to skid logs, mow

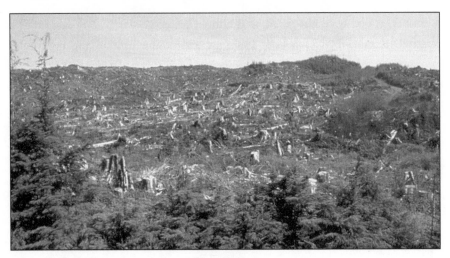

Clear-cut forests between Calais and Cherryfield

hay, pull a dump rake and a dozen other farm and ranch implements. Those were the good ol' days—at least in memory.

歨 歨 歨

A sign caught my eye as I entered the Owls Head Transportation Museum grounds near Rockland: "A *Procyon lotor* crosses here. Please drive slow." At the desk I commented, "You must have a biologist with a dry sense of humor."

"Why's that?"

"That sign about raccoons."

"You're right, but you're the first visitor who has mentioned the sign and knew *Procyon lotor* was the scientific name for raccoon. When our biologist has a few minutes, he sits along the road and chuckles as cars slow and heads swivel left and right trying to see what they are slowing for."

In the museum, a Ford Trimotor airplane built in 1929 caught my eye. As a biologist in the early 1950s, I tossed fifty-pound blocks of salt out the open door of a 1929 Trimotor as we flew over Idaho backcountry. The salt was intended to expand and distribute elk and deer use of the habitat. Instead, my follow-up research showed it concentrated use in small patches around the salt. It turned out to be lousy wildlife management but exciting work.

歨 歨 歨

Astraddle my bike at an intersection in Bath, along the southeast coast of Maine, I was reading a street map when a driver called out, "May I help you?"

"I'm trying to locate a motel for the night," I answered.

After giving directions, he continued, "There's a retired banker in Phippsburg who recently rode his bike from Alaska to Montana. You should talk with him." I called and the bicyclist, Fred Haggett, was eager to tell his story and invited me to stay overnight in his home.

I rode seven miles down the forested peninsula thrusting between the Kennebec River and Casco Bay. Fred was waiting beside the highway. Until 1979 when they built their new home, Fred and his wife, Ada, lived in the McCobb House built by an ancestor of Ada's. The McCobbs or their descendants had owned the house continuously for 200 years before Ada sold it. As I photographed the old but structurally sound and architecturally elegant home, I wondered if houses built today will look this good 200 years from now.

Fred guided me on a bicycle tour of communities along the "peninsular." Webster may think that peninsular is an adjective and peninsula is a noun, but here in Maine they use peninsular as a noun. And they spell it like they pronounce it.

We stopped at Drummond Cemetery where I counted the headstones of fourteen Drummonds buried between 1811 and 1860. Two other tiny cemeteries were within a radius of fifty feet.

"There are eighty to one hundred family cemeteries along this small peninsular," Fred told me.

The next morning, we drove to Bowdoinham where Ralph Purlinger, whom Fred had recommended as a good pilot, had his Piper Super Cub floatplane moored. With me in the front seat, Ralph was ready to provide a floatplane lesson and an opportunity to take photos.

After we taxied to the center of the river, Fred waved us back.

"Your gas tank cap just flew into the river."

"Sonofabitch," Ralph muttered as he crawled out of the backseat and scrambled up the bank to his pickup, screwed off the gas tank cap, returned to the plane, stuck a rag under the cap, and screwed it on—tightly, I hoped.

"C'mon, let's get out of here," barked Ralph as he hopped back in the plane.

Ralph was on the controls with me as we took off. I watched loose metal screws as the cowling in front of me clattered ominously.

Landing on the Kennebec River, I could feel Ralph gently nudging the controls. Rather casually, I thought, he then let me take off and land three times without help. On my first solo takeoff, I wanted to impress him by staying low over the water until we gained enough airspeed for a good climb rate. With droll New England understatement, Ralph's voice came over the intercom, "Better get the nose up or you'll be piloting a submarine." The smooth surface of the Kennebec had totally distorted my depth perception.

🚲 🚲 🚲

From Kittery, in Maine, I biked across the Piscataqua River for a brief coastal traverse of New Hampshire, my second time in that state before leaving New England. Then I rode into Massachusetts, hurrying into a cold wind.

CHAPTER FIVE

Mid-Atlantic Coast

One morn the wind blowed cold and strong, And the leaves went whirling away; The birds prepared for their journey long, that raw and gusty day.

—Henry D. Thoreau

Like Thoreau's birds, I was ready to journey south. Soon I'd be in Boston, near Walden Pond where Thoreau despaired of the world and composed inspirational prose. After moving to his cabin on Walden Pond in 1845, Thoreau wrote: "The water is so transparent that the bottom can easily be discerned at the depth of twenty-five or thirty feet. When I first paddled a boat on Walden, it was completely surrounded by thick and lofty pine and oak woods. Now the dark surrounding woods are gone."

In 1972 Carol and I had visited Walden Pond. We found that Thoreau's lonely cabin was a plain, one-room shanty. We were not prepared for the depressing ugliness of Walden Pond and the decrepit boat and swimming docks, or the decaying bathhouse and shoddy concessionaire stands. Overturned steel drums with open tops spewed garbage on the tiny sand beaches that Thoreau described in such glowing terms. It wasn't worth cycling extra miles to see it again.

I headed into Boston, unsure of my route and concerned about city traffic. My concerns were well founded. A middle-aged cyclist on the Esplanade in Charlesbank Park was having problems, too. Suddenly, two dogs inadequately restrained by their long leashes lunged at his front wheel. Bike and rider sprawled in a heap, with yapping dogs and their screaming lady escort circling him like Indians around a settler's wagon. I stopped and found he needed only calming, not aid.

When I arrived at Howard Johnson's in downtown Boston, the concierge found a room where I could store Old Faithful on the fourth floor. Then he helped us into the elevator.

Elisabeth and I had been talking frequently on the telephone, and she had decided to check on my progress and was flying in from Michigan. I rented a car and met her at Logan International Airport. The next morning we walked the Freedom Trail, discovering two and a half centuries of America's past in such places as the Old Corner Book Store, where Longfellow, Emerson, Hawthorne, and Thoreau used to meet and chat. We also toured the Old South Meeting House, where history engulfed us and it seemed we were there when the Sons of Liberty debated the hated customs laws and later, decided to go to the waterfront and dump the tea as a protest against Britain's tea tax.

After three days in Boston, we began to talk about a possible future together. Then Elisabeth flew home and I resumed my solitary journey.

The ride out of Boston was no better than the ride in. I had been warned that Boston drivers were aggressive and I found it true. Riding through the city was hair-raising, but twenty-one miles after leaving Howard Johnson's I was in beautiful country with dense woodlands and stunning fall colors, and on a curving road with little traffic. I sighed with relief.

After leaving Massachusetts, I wandered through sixty-one miles of quiet Connecticut. Dozens of ivy-covered churches and history-filled cemeteries, small Grandma Moses farms, and country estates sprawled across the countryside. Thousands of road-crossing woolly caterpillars sported patterns of gold, tan, brown, black, and fluorescent orange-red until they were transformed into abstract art by very personal encounters with automobile tires.

I passed hundreds of rocky fields and miles of huge stone walls along the roads. Smaller stone walls, busily partitioning property, zigzagged over the rolling countryside. Yet it appeared the stonemasons never caught up with supply. Thousands of rocks still dotted the landscape.

Mary E. Patenaude, friendly proprietor of the Pomfret Spirit Shop, refused payment for a beer, then gave me her house key, directions to her home a half block away, and instructions for finding the bathroom. Talk about trust!

Later, the couple who ran a crossroads lunch counter, grocery, and gas station weren't as cordial. After I paid for a glass of iced tea, a chair they were refinishing fell off the counter and broke. "Goddamn people come in here and spend a goddamn fifty cents," the man swore. "We ought to close the goddamn place so we can get some goddamn work done."

I walked out, sat on a rock, and enjoyed the peace and quiet while drinking my goddamn fifty-cent tea.

🚲 🚲 🚲

New London, Connecticut, is not a big city, but I sure got fouled up trying to wend my way to the ferry docks. I entered a street where three signs spelled trouble: "Wrong Way," "Do Not Enter," and "Bicycles Prohibited." Escaping, I pushed across a grassy triangle, dodged flower beds, lifted Old Faithful over a fence, and held on as she propelled me down a steep embankment where I found myself on a highway that seemed headed toward the ferry. I hoped so, because the heavy traffic swept me along with little chance to escape. A mile and a half of blaring horns and close calls and I was at the dock awaiting a twenty-mile ferry ride.

Somewhere in Long Island Sound, we crossed into New York state and later docked at Orient Point on the northern coast of Long Island.

Leaving Orient Point, I rode 100 zigzagging miles before finding the city environment I expected throughout the length of Long Island. Instead, I saw Baptist churches and folks walking along the road or riding bicycles. Others were harvesting potatoes, cabbages, corn, watermelons, tomatoes, and zucchini squash. Small stands along the road offered produce for sale. Rows of potatoes grew to the highway's edge. A tractor-drawn potato digger pulled onto the asphalt, spilling potatoes as it turned.

Vineyards flourished in the protection of Little and Great Peconic Bays. Large circular sprinkling systems reminded me of the West and Midwest. Some fields covered 300 acres or more.

Drivers on Long Island pleasantly surprised me. At one point, a taxicab was parked in the bike lane. I swung around, causing a car behind me to slow. As he passed, the driver smiled and waved. Another time, a car pulled up to the highway from a side road. The driver thought the front of his car was in my way so backed up quickly with a big grin.

Of course, there was the driver, who, waiting to cross the street, saw an opening and shot across in front of me. I squeezed my brakes hard, skidding to a stop to avoid the car. Another driver saw this and shook his head in sympathy.

Happily, I didn't encounter any other impatient New York drivers on State Highway 25, known as Middle Country Road. I was having enough trouble as it was. Traffic signs before each intersection read "Right Turn Only," with an arrow for the right-hand lane. At each sign I watched my rearview mirror until there wasn't a car on my tail, signaled a left turn, gritted my teeth, and darted onto the white line between the right turn and straight ahead lanes. All the while, cars zipped past, scant inches on either side of me.

That night, I was the sole camper in the incredible solitude of West Hills Park Campground twenty miles from downtown Manhattan!

After setting up camp in an Adirondack shelter, I walked to the edge of a tree-bordered meadow. Suddenly, I heard the thunder of horse hooves. From the shadows, a white horse with a pale mane and tail flowing galloped across the meadow. In the saddle sat a woman with her blond ponytail shimmering in the spectral moonlight. On the way into West Hills Park, I had biked past a sign pointing to Walt Whitman's home. In *Leaves of Grass*, Whitman wrote, "O the horseman's and horsewoman's joys! The saddle, the gallop, the pressure upon the seat, the air gurgling by the ears and hair."

The scene I had just witnessed seemed, in this place, an appropriate footnote to the day.

Next morning, the air was brisk and clean. Dazzling sunlight flicked across the handlebars as I rolled through Nassau County between stands of pine, hemlock, spruce, and colorful oak. I stopped to ask directions at a Texaco station along Union Turnpike.

Five scruffy-looking fellows were hanging out near the station.

"Ya tryin' to set some kinda record?"

"Where d'ya sleep at night?"

"Carry a gun, don't ya?"

I couldn't believe I answered the last question with, "Nope, I sure don't."

One response wasn't reassuring: "Well, I wouldn't put odds on yer gettin' through New York City with all yer stuff."

A final question: "What d'ya do for entertainment? Get laid once in awhile?"

I considered that a compliment and rode on.

Nine miles later, I hailed an officer in a police car. He stopped in the middle of the street, backing up traffic. Convinced I needed help, he pulled to the curb and looked at my *Guide to the East Coast Bicycle Trail.* Finally he snorted, "That's a poor way to go. Let me show you a better way."

I'd gotten into trouble with "better ways" before. "No thanks," I replied, "I want to follow the recommended bike route."

Exasperated, he said, "Well, follow my rear bumper as close as you can. I'll lead you to Queensboro Bridge." With that, he took off—fast!

When his rearview mirror revealed me as a disappearing speck, he would put on his flashing lights, pull over, and wait for my breathless arrival. For the next three miles, whenever I left too much space, a car would spurt past and dart between us. When this happened the officer would slow, hit his siren and wait until I caught up to his bumpered behind. This was more like the New York I expected—except for this officer's fantastic courtesy.

Stopping on Thirty-fourth Avenue, the black police officer waved me up to his window, looked at my sweaty face, and said, "Sorry I went so fast. This four o'clock traffic across the bridge will be murder. Take care of yourself, and God bless."

The next seven miles were just a blur. I dimly recall the bridge crossing over Roosevelt Island near the middle of the East River. More clearly I recall the hair being sucked away from my left leg by the steady stream of cars thundering past at what seemed only inches away.

I was off the bridge, heading south on Second Avenue, when a twenty-something cyclist with slicked-back black hair came alongside. "How far you ridden that thing?"

"Four thousand six hundred miles."

"You're kiddin'! Where you headin'?"

"The Vanderbilt Hotel."

"That's now the YMCA. Know where it is?"

"Sort of."

"Hey, you'd better let me guide you there. Just follow close and don't let these drivers freak you out."

As we approached Forty-seventh Street, he called over his shoulder, "There she is. See ya!"

With that he shot across the traffic and headed back north. I don't think he heard my heartfelt "Thanks a million."

After I registered at the YMCA and was assigned a room on the ninth floor, the desk clerk saw me struggling to get the loaded bike in the elevator. He ran over to help, then rode up and helped us off the elevator and into the room.

🚲　🚲　🚲

Ann Close, an editor with Alfred A. Knopf had worked with me in publishing my first book a few years ago. We knew each other through correspondence and phone calls but had never met. Ann felt I should write a book about this bicycling adventure and arranged to spend time with me in Manhattan.

She and I took the subway to the tip of Manhattan at Battery Park where I photographed Castle Clinton, built during the battle of 1812. Working back up the peninsula between the East and Hudson Rivers, we visited the U.S. Customs House and Woolworth Building. Later, an elevator took us to the observation deck on the 107th floor of the World Trade Center to marvel at the famous Manhattan skyline. The Chrysler, Pan Am, and Empire State Buildings, and the Rockefeller Center were all within our view. We looked down on Trinity Church at the end of Wall Street. Local wags say it is there to guard the morals of the Financial District. Judging from recent trader scandals, Trinity is failing in its job.

Ann and I spent a second afternoon and evening visiting Chinatown and Little Italy along Canal Street. We enjoyed both evenings in downtown Manhattan without seeing anyone under the influence of alcohol or drugs. Laughing, singing, well-dressed young people packed the sidewalks but never jostled us with their high-spirited antics.

What of the infamous New York taxi drivers? Well, they weren't much affected by red lights but neither were the pedestrians. After Ann took the subway home, I decided to walk back to my hotel. Taxis filled the streets. When the "walk" signal turned green for me, taxis kept zipping through their red light. To test them, I would start into the intersection, raise my arm to show I was going across, and oncoming taxis would skid to a stop.

During my two-mile walk, I never heard a taxi driver use his horn or saw one come dangerously close to pedestrians who must already have known what I discovered by experiment.

After two days in Manhattan, I rode east on Forty-ninth Street to the Waldorf-Astoria for breakfast. No bike rack, so I chained the wheels together and to the frame; then leaned the bike against the front of the Waldorf. Two plain rolls, a small glass of orange juice, and coffee were $6.22. But the maitre d' more than made up for the price. Seeing my cycling attire he asked, "Where is your bike?"

"Out front," I answered.

"Someone will rip it off out there," he warned, and sent two bow-tied waiters out to carry it inside.

As I left the Waldorf and headed south, teenager Eric Perlman pedaled alongside. "Where you going?"

"Staten Island Ferry."

"This is a tough place to ride a bicycle. Let me ride with you."

"I'll signal well in advance," Eric promised as we flowed with Fifth Avenue traffic through Washington Square, then down Broadway to Battery Park at the tip of Manhattan. At the entrance to the ferry station, he explained how to go up an escalator with a loaded bike. "Let the front wheel catch a step, squeeze the front brake. When the back wheel rolls onto a step, squeeze the back brake," he instructed.

To make a painful story mercifully short, I was out of sync in handling the brakes. After losing my grip on both brakes, I and Old Faithful soon resembled a loose cannon on a pitching deck. Seeing my predicament, Eric ran to the bottom of the escalator and helped pull her off. He then made it look easy.

I thanked him and hastily pushed to the turnstile, only to find I hadn't needed to ride the escalator. Flustered, I coasted down a ramp to the automobile entrance for the ferry. An attendant asked, "Ticket, please?" In all the confusion I'd bypassed the ticket office. "Oh, hell," he laughed, "just push your bike on and let's go."

Those heartwarming experiences weren't what I had expected in New York City, just more examples of the unwarranted prejudices I had carried with me.

🚲 🚲 🚲

Memories washed over me as I forged against the wind along Richmond Terrace circling Staten Island toward Goethals Bridge. In early October 1944 I had been temporarily assigned to the Brooklyn Army Base Terminal to help prepare the 75th Infantry Division for shipment overseas. Married only six weeks, I rented a room on Staten Island and called Carol to come and join me. I rode the ferry to Brooklyn each morning. After nine days I was on a troopship, bound for combat in Europe; Carol was on a train, bound for Milwaukee.

Ours had been a single-ring ceremony. On our last night in the lodge, Carol surprised me by slipping a wedding band on my finger. "Will you wear it always?" Now, forty years later, it had never been off my finger.

🚲   🚲   🚲

As I approached Goethals Bridge, a cyclist yelled, "You can't ride in this traffic. You'll have to push your bike across on the walkway." I stopped at the start of the bridge and pondered the problem.

Two police cars were parked on the other side of the divided highway. One policeman signaled for me to stay where I was. Puzzled, I waited as they drove back into town to a crossover, turned, and pulled up beside me. "We wanted to make sure you could get across. If you unpack, we'll put your gear in one squad car, the bike in the other, and take you over."

I felt I could ride it, so thanked them and took off. In the high midsection, with cold winds buffeting me severely, I wished I had accepted their offer.

🚲   🚲   🚲

In Raritan, New Jersey, I bought spiced chicken, spiced cake, and iced tea at Popeye's Chicken, and ate it in my Gateway Motel room. Watching the Detroit Tigers down the San Diego Padres four to one in the final World Series game provided the evening's entertainment.

Exhausted from coping with heavy traffic all day, I fell across the bed and slept until one in the morning. When I awoke, the telephone light was blinking. There had been a call and I had never heard it. The message was that someone had seen me ride in and had called the local newspaper to say that they ought to get a story. I didn't return the call to the newspaper. Instead, I oiled and adjusted the bike and hand-washed socks and shorts. Restless, I read about New Jersey. The state's reputation for corrupt politicians, I found, was as unsavory as its air and water, polluted by smoke-belching, waste-dumping factories and oil refineries. Seven and a half million citizens jammed into New Jersey worried about environmental risks and one of the highest cancer rates in the nation. With these grim facts in mind, I showered and went back to bed for another two hours' sleep.

Next morning, after crossing the Raritan River, I was surprised to find winding roads, smog-free air, deep blue sky, and trees that arched their red and gold-leaved branches across the road. I leaned my bike against the trunk of a huge red oak, then sat on the bank of the Raritan to enjoy the sweet smells of autumn and watch tiny red and gold leaf-boats float down the sparkling clear river. Fields of golden corn, oats, and barley were ready for harvest. Horses grazed in lush pastures behind rail fences. Large barns and silos flanked attractive landscaped homes. No wonder this was called the Garden State.

Across the Delaware River into Pennsylvania, it was cold and the traffic wild as I rode toward King of Prussia. Shortly before reaching Joe and Joann Flather's home, I gave up and called Joe to come and get me. His son, Curt, had been my graduate teaching assistant at Colorado State University.

Early the next morning, Joe and I drove to the Hawk Mountain Sanctuary in the Appalachians of eastern Pennsylvania. Seventy-five years ago, hoards of hunters would have been out on a morning like this. Hunters would often kill a hundred or more magnificent hawks in one day, just for "sport." Many hawks would struggle southward, carrying loads of lead and nursing crippled legs or wings.

Climbing to a rocky promontory, we sat with fifty or so excited, warmly attired men, women, and children armed with binoculars, bird identification manuals, sandwiches, and thermoses of hot coffee. We watched with awe and admiration as sharp-shinned, Cooper's, and broad-winged hawks ascended in thermals created by solar heat from the valleys far below. Others rode the winds deflected from Kittatinny Ridge and continued their migration to southern wintering grounds.

🚲 🚲 🚲

At Honeybrook Restaurant, Sarah served a grilled sticky bun and coffee while telling me that "Gud Kocha Da Hin" on the sign outside was Pennsylvania Dutch for "Good Cooking in Here." She gave me the name of a Mennonite family who might talk with me about their way of life. "But don't expect the Amish or Mennonites to be outgoing toward outsiders," Sarah warned.

When I reached the Stoltzfus farm, Ivan had seen me riding up the lane and stood silently on the front porch as I dismounted. It wasn't until I introduced myself, including name, where I came from, and where I was heading, that a slow smile came to his lips along with the words, "Your trip sounds wonderful. My name is Ivan Stoltzfus. My wife and oldest daughter have gone to a teacher's convention. Because of the convention, school is out and the other children are home today. But come in, we were just getting ready to eat dinner."

Ivan introduced me to his three school-age sons and ten-year-old daughter. Their midday meal featured sandwiches, glasses of cold milk, and rich shoofly pie. When I told Ivan I wanted to see more of Lancaster County, he thought the John Lapp family, who were featured prominently in an April 1984 *National Geographic* story entitled "The Quiet People," would be an ideal family to visit. Without my knowing it, Ivan called the Lapps. "John and Ann Lapp say they will be glad to have you stay with them as long as you like," Ivan reported as he came back into the kitchen where we were eating. He went on, "It's quite a few miles so we'd better let you be on your way. You be sure to come back and stay with us before you leave Lancaster County."

The Lapps' modern dairy barn housed thirty-five Holstein cows. I helped with the evening and morning milking, mostly by putting feed in the mangers, shoveling manure, and staying out of the way. In the 1930s I had worked on a dairy, milking nine cows by hand, but that didn't qualify me to operate the Lapps' state-of-the-art milking equipment.

Supper ended, John and Ann discussed their lifestyle, moral values, and religious convictions. They are Beachy Amish but prefer the term Amish-Mennonites. More liberal than Old Order Amish but stricter than Mennonites, they do not have radio or television but do have electricity and a telephone in the barn. I wondered if the teenagers sneaked out to the barn to call their friends. John and Ann assured me they did not.

Like all the Amish and Mennonites I met, the Lapps didn't go to movies or dances. Neither did they smoke or drink. The many religious groups in Lancaster County seemed to have little else in common. Schisms down through the years produced a variety of attires, appearances, and lifestyles.

I saw gray buggies, black buggies, more stylish buggies. Some folks wore dull gray garb, others wore black. Still others were decked out in more modern clothing. Some women covered their heads with "prayer veilings," others did not. Some men wore full beards, others trimmed them in subtly different styles according to belief. A few were clean shaven.

The Amish folks do not own cars. Some Mennonites drive black cars with all the chrome painted black, earning the nickname "Black Bumper Mennonites." Some homes have electricity, others do not. Some families have telephones in the house; others have none. Still others, like the Lapps, have telephones only in the barn.

In her informative book, *Real People,* A. Martha Denlinger cites such distinctive characteristics and concludes, "These and other differences contribute to the confusion about who's who among the plain folk."

It was nearing midnight when Ann said, "You are sleeping in Geraldine's room." When I started to protest, Ann continued, "She likes to sleep with her sister and this will give her a good excuse." Geraldine's room was large, well decorated, and surprisingly modern except for the big feather bed. It was the first time I had slept in a feather bed since being at my grandmother's house sixty years before. It was just as wonderful as I remembered!

On Friday morning, Calvin, eighteen, and Myma, sixteen, were leaving early to join a group of Amish-Mennonite youths traveling by bus to Albany to sing at two prisons. Later, they would be taken to Niagara Falls as a treat. Although excited about their first big trip, both had to complete chores before

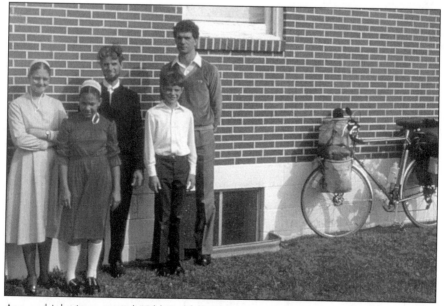

Ann and John Lapp invited "Old Faithful" and me to stay with them and their family during my time in Lancaster County, Pennsylvania.

leaving. Calvin cleaned the barn, and milked and fed the cows. Myma and the other six children had assigned jobs and went at them with gusto. Soon beds were made, breakfast dishes done, kitchen floor scrubbed on hands and knees, and wood floors throughout the huge house dusted and polished. No malingering and no time for complaining.

The Lapp family was so delightful I delayed leaving and didn't reach Intercourse until dark. Tourists may snicker suggestively, but the original meaning honors this name as the place where people gathered for social intercourse. Whether sex occurred was another matter.

In the evening, guests on the Village Tourist Home porch visited, watched firefly lanterns on Amish buggies, and listened to the clip-clop of hooves as young Amish drove into town, apparently only to see and be seen—the Intercourse version of "cruising"?

Saturday night, I returned to the Stoltzfus farm where we visited long into the night about family, lifestyles, and beliefs.

Early Sunday morning, the youngest Stoltzfus boy rode his bicycle several miles with me to meet the rest of the family at Pequea Amish-Mennonite Church. The simple service seemed shorter than the two hours my watch recorded. A wide center aisle separated the women, with their white prayer veilings, from the men. A restless little girl squirmed away from her mother, ran across the aisle, and bounced into her daddy's lap.

After church, nearly fifty men, women, and children surrounded Old Faithful and me, asking questions and inviting us to stay a few more days. But it was time to be moving on.

🚲 🚲 🚲

Beyond the Susquehanna River bridge, a sign greeted me: "Maryland Welcomes You. Please Drive Gently."

The drivers may have been gentle, but commuter traffic into the Baltimore area was brutal. My longtime friend, Stewart Brandborg, however, had invited me to stay a few days in Gaithersburg, and I was eager to get out of the rain and enjoy Anna Vee's good cooking. Brandy and I had been graduate students together thirty-five years before. He studied mountain goats and I studied bighorn sheep in the Salmon River country of Idaho. In 1949, we interrupted a 450-mile horse-packing trip in the backcountry of Idaho so Brandy could marry Anna Vee. Their honeymoon was the final 200 miles of the trip.

Following twenty years with the Wilderness Society, twelve as its executive director, Brandy next spent four years as special assistant to the director of the National Park Service. Now, he was director of the National Leadership Conference sponsored by the ten leading national conservation organizations in Washington, D.C. We had shared many adventures during our years together in Idaho, and I looked forward to visiting with him and Anna Vee.

As I pedaled south along the edge of the narrow, wet shoulder toward Gaithersburg, the wind from a passing RV hurled me over the embankment. A van headed north pulled off on the grass and the young driver ran back, shouting across the highway, "Hey, man, are you okay?"

Wiping mud off my face and spitting gravel, I mumbled, "Yeah, I think so."

"Man, when I saw you cartwheeling down that ditch, I thought for sure you'd need to go to the hospital. You sure you're okay?"

I assured him I was and said I appreciated his concern.

Considering the heavy traffic, steady rain, and my accident, Brandy marveled that I had ridden more than seventy miles and arrived in Gaithersburg with enough energy to celebrate the occasion by jogging a few miles along the C & O Canal with him.

The next day, after driving into Washington, D.C., Brandy, ever the promoter and politician, cajoled our way onto the floor of the Senate, into the halls of Congress, and through the doors of that bastion of old fogies, the Cosmos Club, where we had lunch. While I rested, reminisced, and renewed old friendships, Old Faithful got new gears and chain at a bike shop.

Leaving the Brandborgs, I had pedaled only seven miles south when it began to rain. Soaked and shivering in the cold wind, I boarded White's Ferry to cross the Potomac River into Virginia.

ᗝᖂ   ᗝᖂ   ᗝᖂ

In Fredericksburg, I talked to an old gentleman who was clearing dead limbs from the Confederate Cemetery. He told of a cannonball lodged in some historic building in town. His comment launched an interesting investigation that occupied much of my afternoon.

I asked three yuppie-looking young men about the cannonball. "Never heard of it," said one brusquely as they walked away. An old black man sitting on a nearby bench overheard us. "Whyn't you ast at th' courthouse? Bet they'd know sump'n 'bout it." I left the bike after asking him to watch it for me.

At the courthouse, a lady thought a cannonball was embedded in the ceiling of the courtroom. We went upstairs, unlocked the courtroom, and looked around. Finally, we spotted a bulge. "I think that's it," she said. I was skeptical, but photographed it anyway and thanked her.

When I returned to the bench where I'd left the bike, the old man asked, "Any luck?"

"I don't think so. The lady at the courthouse wasn't too convincing."

"Well, a fren' watched your bike while I went to th' Office of Hist'ry Perservation and ast them. They said th' cannonball is stuck in one a them columns of the ol' Presbyterian church. If you ride yore bike to th' church, I'll walk down and we'll see if it's there."

We did. It was. I photographed it and shook the old man's hand, expressing warm appreciation for his help.

Lee Drive, winding among the rolling, oak-covered hills of Fredericksburg National Military Park, could have been in a Currier and Ives print. Each curve led to more pastoral beauty. Soft sunlight filtered through partially defoliated oaks and maples. Red and gold leaves blended into gilded bronze as they floated gently over the trenches from which Hood, Jackson, and Pickett fought the Union troops.

Though I had read about the Battle of Fredricksburg, I couldn't hear the muskets firing, the cannons booming, and the wounded screaming as Fredricksburg was shelled, looted, burned, and ravaged. That war seemed far away and long ago. I couldn't know the horror of young boys colliding time after time in bloody battles. I couldn't feel what it was like for those 1,500 young soldiers back in the Confederate Cemetery, nor for the 1,600 resting in the Union Cemetery a mile away. But, as an infantryman in four major campaigns in the Pacific and European theaters in World War II, I could appreciate the thoughts of Robert E. Lee as he watched the battle whipsawing across the Shenandoah Valley. When the fog suddenly lifted, Lee peered down on the array of Federal troops and remarked, "It is well that war is so terrible … or we should grow too fond of it."

🚲 🚲 🚲

At a KOA campground, Tom Hughes came over from his tent and invited me to have a martini and meet his wife, Willene, and their bulldog, Percy. They were from Hinsdale, near Chicago, where Tom was principal of two elementary schools and Willene taught science and math. They took a year's leave without pay and were into the fourth month of an adventure planned to take them over much of North America.

Tom, forty-eight years old, told me his mother had died when she was sixty. His dad continued working until he had a stroke, never getting to travel or fulfill his other dreams. Tom and Willene decided not to let that happen to them, and began saving for this odyssey. Tom said, "We'll probably work until we're sixty-five to pay for this, but no one can take the experience away." Good for them!

🚲 🚲 🚲

I pedaled south from Guinea, and suddenly I was in Virginia horse country. Here, just down the road from houses surrounded by small plots of corn, beans, and watermelons grown for survival, the same rich earth produced expanses of greenery for pride, pleasure, and profit. Attractive wooden fences surrounded green pastures where fine Morgan horses and Thoroughbreds frolicked. Elegant homes adorned manicured grounds.

🚲 🚲 🚲

Presquile National Wildlife Refuge is on Turkey Island in the middle of the historic James River. I had called Barry Brady, the manager, and he met the ferry that brought me across. Barry then instructed me how to ride to the refuge headquarters where he lived. Deer season would begin in the morning, so he suggested that this evening would be the best time for a walk.

Several white-tailed deer with magnificent antlers bounded across the path and squadrons of regal Canada geese circled a large field, honking loudly before lowering their gear for graceful landings.

Supper, prepared by bachelor Barry, preceded a pleasant evening when he described experiences on refuges in New York, Hawaii, and Nevada. Afterward, I tossed my foam pad and sleeping bag on the floor and slept without stirring.

🚲 🚲 🚲

On election day I rented a plane at the Chesapeake, Virginia, airport. The air was rough but I felt comfortable controlling the little Cessna while swinging over the Great Dismal Swamp National Wildlife Refuge just north of the North Carolina border. A quarter-mile line of smoke drifted up toward me. The whole swamp seemed to be on fire! Closer reconnaissance showed residues from adjacent soybean fields were burning and smoke was drifting across the swamp.

Gary and Nancy San Julian and their four-year-old son, Eric, had driven to Chesapeake from Raleigh, where Gary is a professor at North Carolina State University. Gary earned his Ph.D. while serving as my graduate teaching assistant at Colorado State University ten years earlier. He and Nancy had befriended my wife, Carol, and son Mark, often inviting them out to dinner during the five months I lived at timberline while photographing the Colorado high country.

While Nancy and Eric explored the countryside by auto, Gary and I spent the next day canoeing in Merchants Millpond State Park in North Carolina. I marveled at the towering bald cypress and tupelo gum trees, draped with luxuriant Spanish moss and resurrection ferns. It was an ecological wonderland. Diverse habitats supported a variety of animal life, from highly poisonous coral snakes and water moccasins to largemouth bass, bluegill, black crappie, and other sport fishes. Raucous waterfowl announced winter as they swooped in from the north. Beaver, mink, and river otter slid down muddy banks into the water. Huge red-bellied turtles, known locally as red sliders, lazed on rocks and logs, watching our canoe glide past.

We divided our time between paddling, photographing, and catching up on each other's lives. Nancy picked us up in the evening and left me at Chesapeake Campground where I had pitched my tent and stored my bike early that morning.

At two in the morning, I shivered out of the sack and pulled on my polypropylene longhandles. Then I slept soundly until awakening at daybreak to find grass, tent, and bicycle covered with frost. It was thirty-one degrees as I crossed into North Carolina wearing the wool jacket, cap, and gloves I had purchased at the L. L. Bean factory before leaving Maine.

ڶ ڶ ڶ

It was a month since I had visited Old South Meeting House in Boston where local citizens decided on December 16, 1773, to go to the waterfront for the Boston Tea Party. Here in Edenton, North Carolina, a group of ladies had a more genteel tea party in the home of Mrs. Elizabeth King on October 25, 1774. Afterward they poured out their tea and vowed not to buy more until Parliament abolished the tea tax. It became known as the Edenton Tea Party, recorded as the first political action by women in this country.

Recently, a writer for *Travel and Leisure* magazine wrote, "Edenton may be the South's prettiest town." I agreed as I biked slowly along Queen and Water Streets, enraptured by the stately beauty of antebellum homes with their wide verandas and huge white columns. There was, however, one discordant note. Alongside these lovely old homes, a Tasty Freeze advertised hot dogs and burgers.

I photographed the cannons contracted by Benjamin Franklin and shipped to Edenton for installation along the bay. Later, federal troops decommissioned them with the observation, "They were of greater danger to the men behind them than to the enemy in front."

🚲   🚲   🚲

The ramshackle grocery in Pinetown was going broke like everything else in town, according to the gray-haired woman who sold me two bottles of orange juice and a package of peanut butter-on-wheat crackers. "All's left are a few farmers and most of them goes to bigger towns to trade," she said. She volunteered that she was a member of Shiloh Free World Baptist Church, one of a half-dozen varieties of Baptists in the vicinity.

When I asked about other denominations she answered, "We don't have no Presbyterians or Methodists or Catholics or such. They're just in the cities, worried more about money than with things of the spirit anyways." I rode on, not in the mood to argue religion "anyways."

🚲   🚲   🚲

Dogs. Yapping, snarling, baying, front-wheel-charging dogs. I'd seen more in the last 200 miles than in the first 5,000. Their voices rose in a threatening crescendo as I pedaled toward New Bern. It reminded me of 1978 when Carol and I were in New Bern while I reviewed wildlife habitat work on nearby Croatan National Forest. Each morning I'd go for a run and soon a coterie of mentally deranged canines would hound my footsteps.

I never was bitten, but the constant harassment annoyed the hell out of me—as it did this morning. Damned if I'd let an untrained, unrestrained, evil-tempered dog interfere with the legitimate exercise of my freedom to enjoy public thoroughfares.

🚲　🚲　🚲

At the Econolodge Motel in Jacksonville, North Carolina, I wrote letters until midnight, then walked into the humid night to clear my head. A security guard, walking his beat, seemed anxious to share problems in his life. I didn't offer counseling, but it seemed he needed a listener. A thirty-nine-year-old marine with a tremendous physique, he supervised physical fitness training at nearby Camp LeJeune. His marine salary didn't provide the income he wanted for his family so he had worked at extra jobs for the past nine years.

We didn't discuss religion, but he quoted scripture that dealt with man as the head of the family. Many were the same passages used by Amish families in Lancaster County, Pennsylvania, to describe their faith. He expressed confusion at events since his wife "became liberated."

"Part of my working at night is for income, but more is to give my wife space without having me around," he explained.

I felt some of his pain as I listened to the intense emotions of this black Hercules who spoke so strongly about his role as husband and father. Then we shook hands and he seemed to feel better for having shared.

🚲　🚲　🚲

I rode southeast from Dixon on State Highway 210 and crossed the arching bridge over the intracoastal waterway to my first experience with barrier islands. For seven miles, from West Onslow Beach to Surf City, I spit sand and witnessed a depressing scene. Junky trailer homes and small houses atop stilts were invading bulldozed openings cut into dunes. Natural cover, such as live oak and yaupon holly, were being cut out, dug up, or pushed aside to make room for cheaply constructed houses.

Down the highway, windblown sand drifted across the road leading to a parking area. Before bulldozers ripped through the sand dunes, American beach grass and sea oats had developed a maze of rhizomes (roots) forming a structural framework like rebar in a concrete abutment. When these sand-stabilizing rhizomes were destroyed, the sandy banks crumbled. The winds took it from there, sweeping the sand into eyes, windshields, homes, and across roads.

When the last major glacial event ended 18,000 years ago and the ice sheets began melting, the sea level rose and has continued rising about one foot every century. That statistic doesn't seem significant until one considers that the slowly rising storm-whipped water along the North Carolina coast eats away an average of three and a half feet of the continent every year. Continuing down the coast, I could hear the awesome power of the Atlantic Ocean chewing on the land.

The most attractive view I photographed along this stretch of beach was a billboard with an artist's rendition of the sun rising over the Atlantic, a silhouetted live oak in the foreground, and three gulls soaring in the blue sky above. It's a helluva note that future generations may have to depend on billboards to know what the natural environment looked like!

At Fort Fisher, I paused at the Civil War Museum to pick up literature and watch an informational movie. When Col. William Lamb took command in 1862, I learned, he didn't like what he saw: only two dozen guns mounted in sand batteries. Over a period of two and a half years while using more than 500 blacks, both slave and free, along with his Confederate soldiers, the colonel created one mile of sea defense and a one-third mile of land defense patterned after the Malakoff Tower fortification in Sevastopol, Russia.

On December 24 and 25, 1864, the Union Army and Navy attacked the Confederate fort but found it too strong and withdrew. What a way to celebrate Christmas!

On January 15, 1865, "after six hours of fierce combat, Fort Fisher was captured by Union forces," according to a brochure. Shortly after this carnage, it was abandoned until restored a century later. Now they make a killing in tourist dollars.

ڲ ڲ ڲ

An eight-mile ferry ride across the windblown white caps of the Fear River estuary brought me to Southport. State Highway 133 led to Yaupon Beach where Buddy Brown lived at the end of Oak Island Bridge. A wondrous assortment of junk, or treasures, depending on your view, filled his shack to overflowing and crept into the surrounding brush. Wedged into this outdoor marvel were rabbit hutches where four females and one male did what rabbits do best, providing Buddy with a high-protein diet.

I found Buddy at the store next door. People in Southport had insisted, "You must meet Buddy, but we warn you that sometimes he won't talk to strangers. Just depends on his mood."

"Hello, Buddy," I began. "Hear you know more about this country than anyone around."

He chewed on his pipe. "Yeah?"

I tried again. "Have time to sit and talk?" He looked at me in silence.

I bought crackers, cheese, and two cold beers. While paying the old man who ran the store, I said loudly, "Well, I'm going to sit on that bench outside and enjoy my lunch."

Ten minutes later Buddy shuffled out to sit on the other end of the bench. For a few minutes he puffed on his pipe while I munched crackers and cheese, and drank beer.

Finally I blurted, "I don't want two beers. You want one?"

"Yeah," he said, reaching out. I sized him up. Small, about five-foot-six, 120 pounds, wiry, with a long, scraggly, graying beard and a clear, sparkling left eye. His right eye was covered with a black patch.

A few minutes later he asked, "Ya got a wife?"

"Did have. She died two years ago."

"Mine died in seventy-five." We sat silently in the humid midday heat. Buddy puffed on his short-stemmed pipe. He shifted and looked at me for the first time. "How old are ya?"

"Sixty-three."

"Humph!" More silence.

"What d'ya do for a livin'?"

"I'm a retired professor."

"Humpfhh!"

After awhile, "Well, I was a shrimper. Fished a forty-nine-foot trawler 'til I couldn't handle 'er alone anymore."

"Couldn't you find someone to go with you?"

"Didn't want nobody. So I sold 'er in sixty-nine an' quit."

Gazing reflectively out toward the Atlantic, Buddy began to talk. He talked about his life as a fisherman, his loves, his triumphs, his tragedies, his lonely night forays out on the Atlantic between Corncake and Shallotte inlets. And he described how the Cape Fear lighthouse often had guided him safely back to the harbor. The sun drained from the sky and became a blood-red crescent in the west.

Landlubber and sailor. Retired professor and retired shrimper. Buddy had weathered many a storm. I hoped I could do as well.

"Now you be careful and write when you get home," Buddy said simply as I sat astride my bicycle, hating to leave.

🚲 🚲 🚲

It was November 15 as I wobbled painfully into South Carolina. I hadn't slept much the damp, cold night before. I woke up nearly every hour to urinate. In the morning, riding forty miles into a headwind had exhausted me, so I stopped a little after noon at the Brookwood Motel in Murrells Inlet, got a room, and laid down to rest. I awoke three hours later soaked with sweat.

Something was wrong.

I showered, put on a dry outfit, and went to the Laundromat with my sweat-soaked clothes. At 8:00 P.M. I returned, totally exhausted, pulled off my clothes, and crawled into bed. Ten hours later I dreamed a snake was sliding across my stomach and slippery worms were crawling off my arms and legs. Arms flailing, I awoke to find the disagreeable creatures were rivulets of sweat running off my body. Bedding and mattress were soaked. After another shower and more dry clothes, I walked shakily to breakfast. That exertion and eating sent sweat streaming down my face and neck.

I decided to stay at the motel for another day.

Weak and shaky all day, I stayed in bed, awaking at three the next morning, drenched in sweat. I took another shower and went back to bed. At six I was streaming sweat again. "Might as well feel miserable on the bike," I muttered. I showered and hit the road.

The seven miles to Litchfield Restaurant were tough. I'd just ordered breakfast when three young people came in. "Is that your bike outside?"

While they asked dozens of questions about my trip, their tiny Volkswagen bug, top-heavy with three surfboards, waited in front.

Before parting they warned me, "Be careful in this country. There are a lot of tough characters around."

Face burning again, I headed for my bike and fresh air.

Bicyclists sometimes stayed at Saint Mary's Catholic Church in Georgetown, I'd been told. Seeking sympathy and a bed for the night, I began, "I've ridden 5,800 miles from Montana and—"

The priest interrupted sarcastically, "Today?"

To this day I don't know why I didn't just go to a motel.

"Do you plan to go to evening mass?" he asked.

I got the connection and responded, "If the sermon isn't going to be too long."

Later, as we walked to church, I said, "You know, you're sure a hardnosed old son of a gun!" The priest just cocked an eyebrow and grinned.

After mass, we returned to the combination rectory/school. I had just thrown my sleeping bag on a cot when the lights went out. Later, I discovered a master locking system had locked the doors from inside and out and the priest had turned the lights off by master switch. I was a prisoner in the dark.

At eleven, the sweating and hourly urination began all over again. Fortunately, I had a flashlight and found the bathroom. I crawled back into the wet sleeping bag after each visit, shaking from the cold. Father had turned off the heat, too. Daylight found me drained in more ways than one.

Exhausted the next morning after pedaling only thirty-three miles, I rested along the highway in Francis Marion National Forest. Later, I started walking along the Swamp Fox Hiking Trail winding through the mixed pine and hardwood forest. It wasn't long until I slipped behind a tree to lose my breakfast.

This wasn't turning out to be a good day.

Five miles of pedaling later my energy disappeared in the face of increasing headwinds. A green lawn in front of a Baptist church looked so inviting that I stopped to eat some cheese, wheat crackers, and a peanut candy bar. Then I stretched out with my helmet as a pillow and rested in the sun.

Another five miles and a red Volkswagen with surfboards atop pulled off onto the grass ahead of me and a woman jumped out. "You don't look like you're feeling so good. We'll take you to our home in Charleston." The surfers I had met in Litchfield Restaurant yesterday morning wanted to rescue me.

"C'mon, we'll pile your panniers on our laps and tie the bike on some-place." A sick cyclist, his bicycle, and gear. Three surfers, three surfboards and their gear, all in a tiny Volkswagen bug? Ah, the optimism of youth. I didn't even want to try. Besides, I was going to complete this trek under my own power or die trying.

Robin was firm. "You have no business out here in this wind. We'll draw you a map to our house in Charleston where you'll stay until you feel better."

All I could say was, "Yes, Mother."

There were times when I wondered if I could fight the wind those last twenty miles. I arrived at Tim and Robin Crump's home a little after six, but my watch didn't begin to tell how long the day had been.

"Have any trouble with the map?" Tim asked.

"Only at that big intersection about a mile back where some teenage boys were playing a game in the street. They looked at the map and told me how to follow your instructions."

"Good Lord! That's one of the toughest black communities in Charleston. Robin and I roll up the car windows and lock the doors when we stop at a stop sign in that area."

"They seemed to like the bike and be genuinely interested when I showed them how I'd fixed the handlebar bag for the camera and tape recorder."

Tim just shook his head. "You're lucky you weren't robbed, beaten, or worse."

I spent another night of copious sweating, frequent jaunts to the bath-room, and parching thirst. Hearing all the commotion, Robin brought dry sheets and a pitcher of ice water in the middle of the night.

Tim made an appointment for me with his doctor. After X rays, poking and prodding, and reading my temperature of 103 degrees, the doctor's evaluation was succinct. "You may have mononucleosis. You have a large tumor in your throat. Your left inguinal hernia needs repair. I suggest you take the next plane home. It will be a long time before you are ready to bike again. You are a very sick man." I rested and sweat the rest of the day.

Next morning, the doctor called Robin and inquired how I was doing. He then asked me to come in for another X ray of my throat. He liked the second X ray even less and advised me to box up the bike, go home, and be happy with having had one heck of an adventure.

I called my son Gary in Atlanta, and he and his wife LaVerne drove to Charleston to pick me up on Thanksgiving Day. Back in Atlanta, Gary called his doctor, who sent me to a clinic for a thyroid scan and ultrasound photos. He didn't like what he saw either. In fact the doctor was so insistent I go home for surgery that he made arrangements from his office for a flight to Denver where I could take a shuttle van to Fort Collins.

The first 5,868 miles had been a terrific experience, and I had no intention of abandoning my goal of circling the United States. But now my timetable would have to change.

CHAPTER SIX

A Stop for Repairs

...every person must accept a certain responsibility for his or her own recovery from disease or disability.
—Rene Dubos, in his introduction to *Anatomy of an Illness* **by Norman Cousins**

Back in Fort Collins, my doctors immediately began a battery of tests to find what ailed me. Bert and Bernice Reid invited me to use their basement bedroom until I was able to hit the road again. Bert had been my supervisor from 1956 until 1965 when I conducted research for the U.S. Forest Service.

My immediate problem was cytomegalo virus, not mononucleosis as suspected by the doctor in Charleston. But his discovery of a thyroid tumor and diagnosis that the hernia needed repair were confirmed. Still, a high fever and astronomical white blood cell count had to be controlled before surgery. Medication and patience were prescribed.

After my temperature leveled at 98.6 degrees, I began bicycling, weight training, and skiing to stay fit and reduce convalescence time later. It also was a time to review and file the books, brochures, maps, pamphlets, and 800 slides I had mailed to my daughter.

After three weeks the white blood cell count had returned to normal and I was ready for surgery.

The scents of antiseptic and clean-scrubbed flesh wafted over me. My eyelids kept drooping. Images of rubber gloves and white masks became blurred. Drowsy, I recognized the voice of Dr. Stan Hensen, who had presided at five of my earlier twelve surgeries.

Seven hours later, it was all over. Still later, the lab report was "Tumor non-malignant," and Stan reported, "The hernia surgery went fine. Take care of yourself and you will soon be back on that bicycle again."

I was dismissed from the hospital on the second day after surgery. The next morning I walked a half mile to mail a letter at the post office. Bert and Bernice were dismayed and suggested I call Dr. Henson "before you do such a thing again."

Stan's response was a laconic: "Fine. Walk as far as you like. Just don't slip and fall in this ice and snow."

That's what I wanted to hear. Within a week I was working out lightly on Nautilus equipment and a stationary bicycle. In three weeks I was flying an airplane, increasing weights and repetitions, and riding a stationary bike an hour at a time.

Though it was good to be back among friends, there were new visions of the future and I wondered if Fort Collins would ever be home again.

Elisabeth flew from Michigan, spent New Year's Eve with me, and accompanied me in my search for a new place to live west of the Rockies, possibly for us both. A week later in Montrose, Colorado, I prepared a bid and made a deposit on seventeen acres with a spectacular view of the San Juan Mountains. An architect friend drew a plan for an earth-sheltered home that would be ideal for the site.

Now that I was feeling stronger every day, inner fires told me to get back on the road again. But not back to Charleston, where I'd have to ride south in summertime heat. I decided San Diego would be a good place to begin about the middle of March. It would be nearly 1,800 miles to Port Townsend near the northwest corner of the United States. Knowing there would be many rainy days, I planned to average only 300 miles a week and get there about May 1. Another six weeks would get me back home to Fort Collins where I could attend mass on Sunday, June 16, in honor of Carol's birthday as originally planned. Of course, this four-month delay meant there would still be over 4,000 miles to pedal before I finished riding the perimeter of the United States. I would wait until mid-October, however, for cooler weather before returning to Charleston to complete the circle.

I called Tim and Robin Crump, my friends in Charleston, and asked them to ship my bike to the Adams Avenue Bicycle Shop in San Diego.

Now I just needed to get in shape so I could ride sixty to eighty miles a day again.

CHAPTER SEVEN

California

Viewed from afar, California is a mysterious, shimmering entity on our continental edge, forever arresting our attention as in bursts of Delphic prescience it hints at what we shall be. Closer up, the power and the wealth (and the pollution) are palpable. There has never been a state even faintly resembling California.

—**Neal R. Pierce and Jerry Hagstrom,**
The Book of America

In June 1984, Frank and Inez Brown had pulled their motor home next to my tent at the International Peace Garden in North Dakota. After an evening of visiting, they invited me to visit them when I reached California. Now, in March of the following year, I accepted their generous offer.

Frank met me at Lindberg Airport when I arrived from Fort Collins and drove me to the Adams Avenue Bicycle Shop for a reunion with Old Faithful. After a mechanic gave her a tune-up, I tested my nerves and bicycle legs by riding through San Diego traffic to Frank's house. Frank handed me a letter that had just arrived from the Realtor in Montrose with whom Elisabeth and I had met in early January. My bid on the seventeen acres where I had planned to build a home had been rejected and the deposit returned. I banked the check and turned my attention and energy to completing the journey.

Next morning, Frank treated me to a day of deep-sea fishing. Retired in 1958, after thirty years in the navy, Frank's favorite recreation was fishing.

My catch for the day was four small ocean bonito. Others on board also caught caloso bass, barracuda, and mackerel.

In a milky blue sky, dollops of white clouds rode a cold wind off the Pacific as Frank and Inez waved good-bye next morning. Frank called out, "Ride careful and keep in touch."

I followed Sports Arena Boulevard across the San Diego River, noticing Sea World to my right. Two miles later, I was on the Bikecentennial Pacific Coast Trail, headed north. It felt good to be back on the road.

A long state, California. There would be 1,114 miles, mostly on State Highways 1 and 101, before I reached the Oregon border. The first night, my neck, hands, arms, shoulders, and legs felt the strain after only forty miles in the saddle. I recalled the time four months earlier when I had arrived in Charleston. Even with a 103-degree fever and after grinding out 62.2 miles on a windy day, I had been in better shape. But I weighed 162 pounds then, 176 now. If I hadn't worked out with aerobics, Nautilus equipment, and a stationary bicycle after surgery, my body would have been in even worse shape.

I pitched my tent in South Carlsbad State Beach Campground, took a cold shower, and was in my sleeping bag before dark. The surf pounding the beach seemed to massage my tired body and I slept soundly.

Next morning, I realized that not only my body but also my bike needed attention. Less than a mile from the campground, the loaded front rack loosened and fell on the front wheel. A bungee cord made temporary repairs. After climbing a couple of hills, missing a couple of downshifts, and having the chain fly off the gears each time, I decided serious repairs would be better than greasy hands and skinned knuckles. I returned to Carlsbad where I had seen a bike shop.

At the Pacific Coast Cycle Shop, Don Brokenshire replaced the badly worn thirteen-, fifteen-, twenty-one-, and twenty-six-tooth freewheel cogs and installed a new Shimano Uniglide chain. Astride a more smoothly operating bike, I headed north again. But this wasn't to be my day. A mile past San Onofre Nuclear Power Plant, I belatedly spotted glass strewn across the bike path. More time out while I patched the front tire.

Two days later, I reached Peter Joslyn's home in El Segundo. I had met Peter in Minnesota the previous July. Now I called from Peter's house to rent a Cessna 172 and hire an instructor at Torrance Airport. Later, while Peter pointed out local landmarks, we flew over Marina Del Rey, Redondo Beach,

Palos Verdes, San Pedros, and Long Beach. We looked down on Marineland and Terminal Island Prison and peeked into backyard swimming pools of the affluent in Torrance. Then we flew along the beach and Esplanade where I would bike the next day.

Before returning to the airport, I swung into position for a final wide-angle photo showing the bay area from the Pacific to the San Bernardino Mountains. But the peaceful euphoria of flying 2,000 feet above the cities was replaced by harsh reality when I returned to the Los Angeles Traffic Control Area and called Torrance Tower.

"Cessna five-five-one-two-six, over Queen Mary at two thousand feet, inbound, landing with Information Bravo." I had reviewed procedures and thought smugly how professional I sounded, but there was little time for self-congratulation. Torrance Tower answered, "Cessna five-five-one-two-six, fly heading of two-sixty and squawk one-fourteen-point-six."

Do what? I vaguely remembered reading about "squawking." Fighting for time I responded, "One-twenty-six, say again?"

"Set your transponder to one-fourteen-point-six and squawk immediately." I dialed 114.6 on the transponder. But squawk? Then I remembered. That little button far right on the instrument panel sends a signal enabling radar to pick me up. With Cessna 55126 now identified, the rest should be a piece of cake.

It wasn't. About all I recall was a flurry of instructions such as, "Report over Thomas Bridge." Then, "Turn to heading of two-ninety, descend, maintain 1,500 feet, and report over Union Refinery," quickly followed by, "Watch for a Bonanza at two o'clock, altitude unknown."

My mind asked, "What's all this about?" My mouth curtly acknowledged, "One-twenty-six."

Very professional. Though I sure as hell didn't know what I was doing, except I understood the last transmission and looked wildly for a Bonanza at "altitude unknown"!

The controller directed me to descend rapidly from an altitude of 1,500 feet over the Union Refinery to 100 feet over the end of runway 29R. I couldn't believe how much I had to pull back the throttle and extend the flaps to descend fast enough. In the mile-high air of Colorado, you drop like a rock. Here I seemed to float forever. As wheels touched pavement, I breathed a sigh of relief.

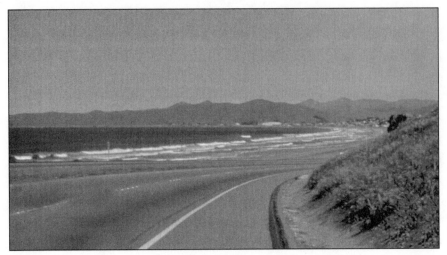

Southern California Highway 101 runs along the picturesque Pacific Ocean.

In all this the instructor, a laid-back sort of fellow, offered only a few terse comments. Undoubtedly, though, his hands and feet were close to the controls, ready to avoid total disaster.

There was no floating the next day as I struggled on my bike against head-winds for sixty-two miles. After Peter had mentioned the dangerous characters I might meet in beach restrooms and described the complex mix of bike paths, city streets, and heavily trafficked Coast Highway that lay ahead, I quickly accepted his offer to ride with me through the worst of it.

After nine miles we had passed the famous-for-fishing Washington Street Pier and scanned graffiti on walls along Venice Beach. Two miles farther north, we were in a different world at Ocean Park where I photographed costly high-rise apartments.

I said goodbye to Peter in Santa Monica and headed north. "Watch out for glass and nails on the bike path," he warned. "When you get on the Pacific Coast Highway, just tighten your helmet and go for it!"

North of Malibu, a sign surprised me with the information that I was leaving Los Angeles County. I checked my bike maps again. In the 100 miles from San Clemente to Malibu, the name "Los Angeles" didn't appear on my bicycling maps. Incredulous, I realized I was already north of the city.

🚲   🚲   🚲

My concerns about riding through Los Angeles reminded me of the spring of 1952 when I had equipped an army surplus seven-foot rubber raft with oarlocks and made a fifty-mile solo float trip down the Middle Fork of the Salmon River in Idaho. I was apprehensive about the Aparejo Rapids, which were rated Class 3, quite dangerous. I had only been through them once when I manned the rear sweep of a twelve-man rubber raft while veteran boatman Red Smothers handled the front sweep. About all I recalled seeing as we careened through the rapids were huge boulders, foaming water, and Red's backside. Remembering there were several small rapids before reaching Aparejo Point, I worried a little about being able to recognize the "big one."

Sooner than expected I picked up speed and began rowing furiously to navigate the main channel, stay off boulders, and keep from capsizing. "Man," I thought, "that was a rough sucker. I wonder what Aparejo will be like?" Finally in calmer water, I saw two backpackers on the trail beside the river and called out, "How far is it to Aparejo Rapids?"

"You just came through it," one fellow said with a grin.

♾ ♾ ♾

Now, finding I had already passed Los Angeles, I felt similar relief. The worst was over.

In Huenema that night, a margarita followed by a rich clam chowder self-served from a large crock centered on my table revived me enough to toss my own salad from a cart wheeled in by the attentive waitress. Tender T-bone, baked potato, and garlic bread brought about full recovery. Every few minutes the busboy checked my water glass and took away empty dishes. All this for $11.49, including gratuity!

The clientele appeared to be working class. Many of the men were big and barrel-chested, often big-bellied. Most wore sweaters or turtlenecks. Many women were large, dark-skinned, and attractive. Loud, good-natured voices and boisterous laughter drifted in from the bar, along with a handsome fellow in a cardigan. Sticking out a huge paw, he boomed, *"¡Alo! ¿Como estas? Me llamo Carlos."* Then Carlos moved easily into fairly good English. "I see you at the motel with your leetle bike. Where you goin'?"

Carlos was so effusively friendly I wound up revealing my full itinerary—past, present, and future.

"*¡Caramba!* You crazee?" he exploded.

Now it was my turn. "Who are these people?"

"Most are Costa Ricans or Puerto Ricans. We're carpenters and painters and plumbers and electricians." Later he added, "We like good times after work."

Moving away, Carlos beamed, "*¡Buena suerte! ¡Que Dios le bendiga!*"

Noting my puzzled expression, the manager offered, "He says, 'Good luck and God bless.'"

Next morning at Denny's, a man about my age came to my table. "Name's Norman Batten. Saw you ride up. I'd like to buy your breakfast."

As we settled into a booth, Norman told me, "I've lived in this area all my life. Most of the time I've been in the car business, primarily auto repair. It's been a good life. I have a wife, five children, and scads of grandchildren. Most live nearby. We don't travel a lot. I got that out of my system as a paratrooper in World War II."

"But," Norman continued, "my wife and I go to symphonies, operas, and theater productions from Los Angeles to Santa Barbara. We are small town and rural here in Ventura County, but the county is becoming a cultural center and we can't think of a place we'd rather live."

As the waitress kept our coffee cups full, I was delighted to find that Norman was also enthusiastic about nature and well informed about land use.

"Years ago," Norman told me, "soils in Santa Clara valley were fertile and thirty feet deep. Intensive farming has cost us most of that. Salty water from high tides and storms comes in, but the rivers used to flood periodically and flush the salt back to the ocean. Now most coastal rivers are so controlled by dams that floods don't occur. The soil is getting so salty that farm production is declining.

"The Santa Clara River seldom flows anymore," Norman went on. "Estuaries, once filled with wildlife, are dying because not enough freshwater flows from the coastal mountains to mix with the salt water and maintain them."

"I'm surprised," I told Norman. "I wouldn't think a man in the auto repair business would know so much about farming and ecology."

"Well, many of my customers are farmers. And I care about our environment. I've fished in most of the canyons along the coast since I was a kid. Used to see lots of black bears and condors in every canyon. Every once in a while I'd see a mountain lion or its tracks."

"Do you still get up in those canyons?"

"No. Even if I had time, dams now block most of them," Norman complained. "Some bears are still around, but there aren't many mountain lions, and the California condor is nearly extinct. There's just too much development of all kinds.

"You've just passed the offshore island of Anacapa," Norman went on as the waitress warmed up our coffee again. "It once was an important nesting ground for brown pelicans. In the 1960s, Montrose Chemical Company of Los Angeles flushed DDT storage tanks with seawater assuming the amounts of the chemical washed into coastal waters was insignificant. But the DDT concentrated in anchovies eaten by pelicans. This caused thinning of pelican eggshells. As a result, only one egg hatched in more than 500 nests in 1970, and the California brown pelican population almost disappeared."

Norman had more. "Public pressure and new laws caused Montrose Chemical to stop dumping DDT-contaminated waste. In only a few years the pelican population has come back in a big way. If we just put our knowledge to use, we can do a lot to improve our environment."

Pedaling toward Santa Barbara, I thought about the people I'd met on this trip. Many totally ignored me. Others came across as, "What the hell's he doing with that bicycle on *my* highway?" Still others were curious. "Why would you ever want to do a thing like this?"

Then there were people like Norman. Knowledgeable about many subjects. Enthusiastic. Interested in the rest of the world and its diverse people. I'll bet he was a top-notch car repairman, too.

Twenty miles north of Port Hueneme, an elongated pullout overlooked the ocean. I stopped to investigate. It was a self-serve parking meter zone reserved for RVs. The pullout was several hundred yards long, white-lined neatly into fifteen-by-forty-foot rectangles. Motor homes, parked at the back of each rectangle, left a short, partitioned beachfront plaza. At one hundred-yard intervals there was a parking meter box, a dumpster, and portable toilets.

There was no one in sight, so I walked in front of the motor homes to get a feel of why people parked here. People were in each motor home, doors open, with TVs, radios, or tape players blaring.

I wandered down to a big rock near the ocean to eat lunch and watch the surf. In seeming defiance of the laws of physics, huge rollers came thundering in, only to tear themselves apart, squandering their energy and managing only a modest climb up the beach. Smaller waves quietly crept in to lap at the base of my rock, proof that grandiosity isn't essential to accomplishment.

I wondered about these urban escapists. Why did they sit inside while roaring trucks shook their motor homes and drowned out their blaring audio equipment? Tourists bring the city with them as they escape smog and congestion to park just a few feet off the highway, and then let raucous music drown out the soothing sounds of the surf.

A hundred yards away on my rock, soft sunlight warmed my back, scented sea breezes wafted away my sweat, seabirds called, and the resounding surf muted the man-made noises.

🚲 🚲 🚲

Climbing 918-foot Gaviota Pass was the first time I'd been more than a hundred feet above the ocean since leaving San Diego. Realizing my legs still needed conditioning, I crossed the pass and coasted into a dazzling valley with the magnificent Sierra Madre Mountains in the background. After coexisting for hundreds of miles with traffic that ranged from heavy to horrendous, this was paradise!

Savannalike stands of scattered oak surrounded pastures where Hereford and Angus cattle, and fine-looking race and saddle horses grazed. I passed the Alisal Guest Ranch, with its rodeo grounds, tennis courts surrounded by umbrella-shaded tables, and a golf course, all overlooked by a luxurious home atop a bluff. In the quaint but touristy village of Solvang, a couple inside Ellen's Pancake House smiled as I locked my bike in front of the window. When I walked in they motioned me to join them.

Don Sharpe, an architect, had just completed a new home near El Capitan State Beach for his new wife, Kaye. She was seven months pregnant and pleased to be settling down after vagabonding around the country alone on a motorcycle. We talked about the spectacular mountain towns of Ouray, Montrose, Gunnison, and Crested Butte where Kaye had ridden in Colorado.

Don told me I would pass several wineries in the Sisquoc River valley before reaching Santa Maria. "Many are owned by doctors or other professionals who bought them for tax write-off purposes," he explained.

At an Exxon station in Santa Maria, the attendant directed me to Motel 6. Next morning, the lively caroling of songbirds outside the motel window awakened me. After eight o'clock mass, a breakfast in the parish hall offered all the pancakes, eggs, ham, and coffee I could stow away for $2.50. Two elderly couples sat at my table.

"Where do you stay at night?"

"Mostly in campgrounds along the beach."

"Carry a gun?"

"Don't need one."

"Well, you've just been lucky. A lot of weirdos stay in those beach campgrounds. You'll be going through Guadalupe later this morning. Be careful. A lot of mean Mexicans are up there."

As I rode through Guadalupe, dark faces broke into broad smiles and friendly hands waved vigorously. No occasion to return gunfire, even if I had carried a gun.

🚲 🚲 🚲

My main recollection of San Luis Obispo involves two kinds of nourishment: a fondue dinner with Chardonnay at Wine Street Inn and spiritual food after riding up a hill to Mission San Luis Obispo de Tolosa. Established in 1772, San Luis Obispo is one of the earliest of twenty-one Spanish missions in California. As I approached, a choir was practicing and clarion young voices floated down from the hilltop in the soft evening air. Enthralled, I sat outside and listened as dusk enveloped the quaint Spanish church.

Early the next morning I enjoyed the landscape of interspersed vineyards and orchards and tried, unsuccessfully, to ignore the garish billboards advertising the William Hearst Castle. Signs informed me "the castle has 100 rooms, including thirty-eight bedrooms, a movie theater, a billiard room, two libraries, and a vast medieval dining hall with carvings of saints on the ceiling." I wondered what the saints thought as they looked down on this extravagant opulence.

Later, I topped a hill to gasp at the breathtaking beauty of the blue Pacific, featuring dome-shaped Morro Rock in the foreground. This huge monolith, called the Gibraltar of the Pacific, seems a symbol of security. But sharing this spectacular landscape were three huge smokestacks rising above the highly controversial Morro Bay Nuclear Plant. Not my idea of security symbols.

By midafternoon fierce headwinds held me to three miles per hour and nearly yanked the handlebars from my control near San Simeon State Beach Campground. I pulled in and fought the wind to pitch my tent behind a clump of shrubs. Sweating mightily, I locked my bike to a picnic table and looked for a restroom with showers. There were only portable toilets and a nearby standpipe with a faucet. Seeing no one I leaned into a howling wind and stripped for a hasty scrub down in icy water. Then I dove, naked, into my tent. Finally snug in my sleeping bag, I remembered a hauntingly similar incident forty-two years earlier.

🚲 🚲 🚲

The 37th Infantry Battalion had landed on Amchitka far down the Aleutian Chain in howling winds on the twelfth of January 1943. Our transport ship, the *President Cleveland,* partially sank just off shore. We scrambled over the side on rope ladders into landing craft that couldn't quite make it to shore because of the storm. We jumped, armpit deep, into the icy Bering Sea and waded ashore.

I was in one of the squads dispatched to scout for Japanese troops supposedly on the island. But our only adversaries were the weather and the U.S. Army, which had shipped our arctic footgear to the South Pacific. We wore leather combat boots in knee-deep wet snow. Carrying full combat gear, we walked from dawn to dark, stopping every hour to pull off our boots, pour out icy water, wring out socks, put them back on, and begin walking before our feet froze.

On the second night we camped near the base of a small cliff on the beach. Eleven exhausted soldiers immediately set up tents and shivered into their sleeping bags, wet clothes and all.

I opted to stay up. Though covered with snow, piles of driftwood yielded dry pieces of fuel. Soon I had a roaring fire going and began scavenging the beach. I was surprised to find a large kettle and some wire. Later I found a freshwater spring near the base of a cliff.

With driftwood and the wire I built a tripod and hung the kettle of water over the fire. Next I wired together a drying rack. Then I peeled off my wet clothes and hung them on the rack. When the water was hot, I took my first freshwater bath in weeks.

For a couple of hours, I stood naked beside the fire, turning frequently to avoid scorching one side or freezing the other, and moving clothes so they would dry, not burn. When the fire dwindled, I would "streak" up the beach to get more driftwood.

In the meantime, my squad members were wet, cold, miserable, and slept very little. Next morning I was dry, clean, and felt much better than my companions, though I hadn't lain down or gotten a wink of sleep.

                                                                        椖 椖 椖

At sunrise on March 25, 1985, the tent, bicycle, and picnic table were white with frost. I was trying to deice my outfit when a rugged old cattleman walked over from his camper to supervise and to tell me he had seen it a lot colder this time of year. Maybe so but it was plenty cold for me as ice particles adhered so tightly to the tent that I finally rolled it up, ice and all, and packed it on my bike.

Midmorning I turned off the highway where a sign pointed to the San Simeon Beach Post Office. There, the postmaster volunteered, "The ninety miles to Monterey will be the worst biking you'll find anywhere in the United States. The highway has no shoulders. There are dozens of steep hills. Drivers are fast and hostile. Be careful in Gorda. Some of the toughest characters along the coast hang around there."

After a few miles, headwinds brought torrential rains that lasted the rest of the day. I donned my Gortex and soon was drenched with rainwater and sweat. Finally, I stripped to my biking shorts and T-shirt and rode in the pouring rain to Gorda.

"Gorda," Bobby Johnson told me over a cup of coffee in Sorta Gorda Restaurant, "means fat-assed woman." Later, I looked it up in a Spanish dictionary. Sure enough, *gorda* is feminine gender for "fat." Bobby's interpretation may not have been precise but probably reflected what the Spaniards had in mind when they named the place.

"Gorda has two industries, jade and marijuana," Bobby said. "They used to mine for jade back in the mountains. More recently they dive for it, mostly in Jade Cove north of here. This is the only place in the world where Pacific blue jade is found. They also find blue-green nephrite jade."

Less forthcoming about marijuana, Bobby continued, "There's a lot of it grown around here and a lot of people used to make $100,000 or more a year. You'd see rolls of hundred-dollar bills pulled out by people who carried a sawed-off shotgun in their pickup trucks."

"What happened?" I asked.

"Coast Guard helicopter surveillance put an end to a good business. Not much money around here now."

I had a huge dinner as rain crashed against the window and water poured down the roadside ditch until it overflowed across the highway. I needed a dry place to spend the night. Bobby offered his small camper, balanced under some trees on the mountainside. For ten bucks he had a deal.

I paid my bill and asked the waitress for a tea bag to take to the camper. The dour restaurant manager, who had been eyeing me suspiciously, called out, "Charge him sixty cents plus tax for the tea bag." With the Coast Guard nosing around, Gorda's economy was tough!

I settled into my hillside hideaway. Plastic bags inside the panniers had kept clothes and other items dry. But when I turned the panniers upside down, water poured out onto the floor. The ground cloth, tarp, and tent, covered with ice when I packed this morning, dripped in the tiny bathroom where I stretched them out as best I could. Before getting too cozy, I went back into the rain, found a dry spot under the porch of an abandoned house, dragged in my bike, and crouching under the porch, wiped it dry and applied oil to its vital parts.

Back in the camper I toweled down and put on dry clothes. There was a tap on the door. Bobby stood outside with beer and a hankering to visit. It was a slow day in Gorda.

After Bobby left I had the propane stove going full blast and my tiny quarters were steaming from drying clothes and gear. I decided to stock up on a few supplies at the grocery store. There, locals were talking of eighty-mile-per-hour gales south of San Francisco and forecast of a two-day storm. I realized I might be in Gorda longer than expected so I began reflecting about riding along the coast.

I'd been on the road twelve days, but traveled only 470 miles. Five months ago, I was cycling sixty to eighty miles a day down the Atlantic coast—of course, I was fourteen pounds heavier now. Perhaps, too, there were lingering effects from my two surgeries.

After leaving San Diego, I'd followed the Bikecentennial Pacific Coast Trail, sometimes on the shore-hugging esplanade, sometimes on narrow shoulders of State Highway 1 or U.S. 101, and sometimes on special ten-foot-wide north and south bike lanes separated by a yellow line. Joggers, race walkers, and just plain walkers far outnumbered bicyclists on the trail for the first 100 miles north of San Diego. North from San Clemente, though, hundreds of cyclists were streaming both north and south.

The beach pays a price for this heavy recreational use. California Parks and Recreation employees, riding three-wheeled bicycles that carried shovels, rakes, and brooms, were sweeping sand and debris off the trail. In Mission Beach a man told me, "The bulldozers you asked about are scraping last week's filth into piles. Trucks will haul the stuff someplace. People around here behave like animals."

A few miles farther on I passed tennis courts near the beach and rode along the base of ocean cliffs while gawking at extravagant homes such as one formerly owned by actor Charles Laughton. I'd be uneasy living up there. Earth slides had swept into the bike path every quarter to half mile for several miles, forcing me to ride around them.

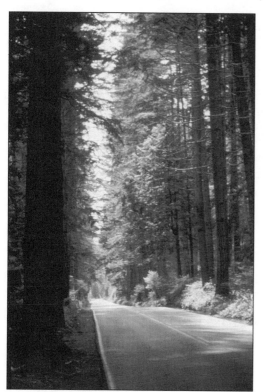

My first twenty miles out of Gorda were misty but pleasant. Then, ahead, I saw sheets of water slanting downward. I rode to Pfeiffer Big Sur Campground in a downpour. I had covered my panniers and top-loaded gear with plastic trash bags so I had a dry sleeping bag in a dry tent pitched on a deep bed of dry needles under a huge redwood tree that night. But it rained all night and water seeped into the tent. Wet again!

Giant Redwoods along U.S. 101 in California

Ben Martin had been a sergeant in my command through World War II campaigns in France, Belgium, and Germany. Our only contacts since then had been Christmas letters. Now, I called and he invited me to stay with him and his wife, Charlotte. Ben suggested they meet me in Half Moon Bay, but he became anxious and started down State Highway 1 where they met me eight miles south of town. It surprised us both, I think, to find ourselves in each other's arms with tears flowing down our cheeks. Hardly our image of two old combat soldiers!

Ben loaded the panniers and all my gear in their car so I could enjoy a fifty-pounds-lighter ride. In Half Moon Bay, firemen let me store my bicycle in the firehouse while Ben and Charlotte took me to their home in Castro Valley.

After we had rewon the war, a nostalgic day wasn't enough time to catch up on our lives since we had last seen each other in Europe in 1945 ... but we tried. Dinner with one of my ex-graduate students, now a U.S. Forest Service employee in California, rounded out the day nicely.

After two days with Ben and Charlotte, I retrieved Old Faithful from the firehouse and pedaled north again.

Construction work on the Golden Gate Bridge prohibited riding across on my bicycle. Instead, a van pulling a flatbed trailer was provided to transport cyclists and bikes across. When we reached the north end of the bridge, Virgilio Hoffman, who also crossed with his bike, saw me struggling to get my loaded bike off the trailer and came over to help.

Virgilio, a merchant seaman from Chili, had lived in San Francisco for twenty-two years. He kept a room in a cheap hotel where he left his bicycle while at sea, mostly sailing to the Orient. He enjoyed biking whenever possible. He said it was easy to get confused in this area, then rode with me on some disjointed bike paths to Mill Valley. From there, I made it to a motel in San Anselmo, getting lost only once.

ᗷᗙᗤ ᗷᗙᗤ ᗷᗙᗤ

"You're one hell of a bicyclist. Saw you before that long hill back there and tried to catch up. Even with your heavy load you kept pulling away." I liked Dick Bricker immediately.

At the Cheese Factory on a back road about twenty miles north of San Anselmo, we became acquainted over fresh French bread, cheese, and wine.

Dick was a bomber pilot in World War II. After leaving the air force, he spent years in sales and administration with IBM. Now retired, he worked with young people with learning disabilities. His insights were interesting and reassuring.

"We don't have enough faith in the abilities and toughness of our youngsters today," Dick asserted. "You and I grew up in the depression years. We worked hard. We went off to war for three or four years. We came back and life gradually became easier. We had children and wanted to protect them from the hard life we had."

He continued, "Adults now think it's a hardship if kids walk or ride a bike a mile to school or to a Little League game, so we drive them. We acquiesce, or often help, as they get their first set of wheels. We see to it they have as big a TV set as the neighbor kids. We don't have the guts to say 'no' when their natural energies and enthusiasms for learning and physical challenges wane in front of the boob tube.

"But the more I work with these kids," Dick asserted, "the more I'm convinced they can far exceed our expectations. They need our support and guidance. But more, they need us to have faith that given the chance, they will come through for us."

I agreed. Leaving Dick, I turned inland to Santa Rosa and the home of Marge and Bill Bush. Before World War II, I had dated Marge at the University of Idaho.

"Remember those dance programs you fellows used to fill out before our dances?" Marge asked as we sat in the hot tub with margaritas close at hand. "We were so formal."

"Yeah," I remembered. "We always reserved the first dance, last one before intermission, first one afterward, and last dance of the evening for our date. We traded some or all of the other dances. You danced with his girl, he danced with yours. It was great."

"Sure," Marge retorted. "You guys traded us like property."

"Not really," I defended the good old days. "But you should have heard our discussions of each other's dates as we set up the programs. Hints on what to talk about, what jokes you'd tolerate, how tight we could hold you while dancing cheek-to-cheek, if you had cute friends, if you … "

Marge picked up the reminiscing: "Remember those crisp fall days in forty-one, just before Pearl Harbor? We'd take long walks, then come to the student union where we'd drink hot chocolate or coffee, turn on the jukebox and dance cheek-to-cheek to 'In the Mood.' Or we might jitterbug to 'Tuxedo Junction,' fox-trot to most anything by Tommy Dorsey or Artie Shaw, or waltz to romantic music by Vaughn Monroe."

Bill sipped his drink and listened in amused silence. He had known Marge in high school but wasn't at the University of Idaho before the war. In 1945, before returning for a second tour of sea duty as a navy pilot, Bill had married Marge. After the war, he returned to the University of Idaho where he and I became acquainted and Marge met Carol. Bill then earned a master's degree in chemistry and worked for thirty-two years as a successful chemist with Shell Chemical Company before retiring.

After enjoying their gracious hospitality for two days, I rolled across the sensors that opened the steel gate to let me leave their exclusive Wild Oak Private Residential Community.

A couple of days later, U.S. 101 led me north toward the famous California redwood stands. The first evidence of what chambers of commerce like to call The Redwood Empire was the Boise Cascade redwood sawmill at Healdsburg and trucks loaded with redwood logs rumbling down the highway.

I had scarcely penetrated the natural beauty of a redwood grove when a gaudy sign trumpeted "World Famous Tree House." After riding 162 miles from the Tree House through scattered stands of redwoods, I photographed another huge sign: "Trees of Mystery. Klamath, California." Nearby, I photographed thirty-foot statues of Paul Bunyon and his blue ox surrounded by manicured hedges and formal flower gardens. Beyond these were scraggly trees remaining after the virgin redwoods had been logged.

The thirty-two-mile Avenue of the Giants wound in and out of dozens of memorial redwood groves that shared space with gift shops, motels and restaurants, and numerous novelty shops built on intervening private lands featuring redwood and driftwood products.

At the Immortal Tree a large sign proclaimed: "Estimated age of this large redwood tree is 950 years. It has survived lightning which removed the top, the loggers axe in 1908, and the forest fire and flood of 1964. Original height of the redwood was 298 feet and now stands at 248 feet. The diameter at the base is 14.5 feet and three feet at the top. Total volume of boardfeet in this tree is 104,380 which would build several homes."

It would, too, if loggers had their way.

Also along those thirty-two miles where the highway partnered with the winding and milky Eel River, were the towns of Phillipsville (population 250), Miranda (population 350), and Redcrest (population 350). I passed a half mile of unpainted shacks, sheds, and trailers; rusted, junked cars; sheep, chickens, and peacocks; and decrepit fruit and vegetable stands with signs announcing "Produce Organically Grown."

From the map, I assumed the next place was Pepperwood but no sign documented the blame.

Yes, there were unsightly places like this and too many gaudy tourist traps. Yet, while in a redwood grove earlier on Easter morning, I had taped: "Gigantic trees. Majestic. Awe-inspiring. The three-part harmony sung by the choir of thrushes, warblers, and vireos is lovely. Shafts of misty early morning sunlight create stained-glass windows in this glorious cathedral."

Later, at Saint Joseph's church, the twenty-person choir sang praises to the Lord with great gusto. I lingered to visit with parishioners after mass. It was good to be there. I'd almost given up hope of finding a church and Easter services.

🚲 🚲 🚲

"Dwight Smith!" shouted a lady as she ran across the Motel 6 parking lot in Arcata. Blinded by the setting sun as she planted a kiss on my cheek, I thought, "nice" while wondering, "Who in hell is this?" Then Percy came around the corner of the motel and I knew. Percy was a bowlegged bulldog I had met last Halloween night in a KOA campground near Fredricksburg, Virginia, along with his owners, Tom and Willene Hughes. I could hardly believe our paths had crossed again a half year later on the opposite side of the continent.

Since that October, they had continued their quest to see North America. "We've bought a motorcycle and little trailer since you saw us," Tom reported. "It's fun and gives us more mobility to search out interesting places."

At dinner that evening, Willene said, "There's so much to catch up on. Let's eat breakfast together tomorrow."

After breakfast at McDonalds, I said goodbye to Tom and Willene, and headed for the bathroom, *always* my last act before hitting the road. When I stepped out of the restaurant, I heard Tom exclaim to a man he was talking to out front. "I can't believe this, but that's him all right!"

Jon Hooper had just driven up and thought he recognized me visiting inside with Tom and Willene. Jon was my graduate teaching assistant in 1972. We hadn't seen each other since 1974. By the time we reconnected, he had become a professor at Chico State and was returning from working with his graduate students on a project up the coast. We all went inside for more coffee and visiting and a very late morning start for me. But what delightful coincidences.

🚲　🚲　🚲

Bright red tam-o'-shanter cocked rakishly on his head, a tan, trim man called out, "When you've finished showering, come over for a port and brandy." I had pitched my tent in Prairie Creek Redwood State Park within shouting distance of this fellow's Delta motor home and was heading for the restroom with a towel around my neck and change of clothes over my arm. An ordained Catholic priest, Ward Bowling, wearer of the tam, had spent thirty years as an air force chaplain before retiring to Santa Monica where he lived with his sister. When we met, he was spending much of his time in his motor home enjoying the beauties of nature and golf courses throughout the country.

Ward was getting ready for a tournament in Ontario, where he planned to enter both Senior and Open Divisions. During his air force career, he had entered golf tournaments all over the world. A civilian pilot before priesthood, Ward had tried to talk the air force into teaching him to fly fighter planes, not for combat but to improve his rapport with other pilots in the squadron.

There was another side to Ward Bowling. As we talked into darkness, he set two candles on the table. Before he closed the door, moths flew in, attracted to the flames. Ward spent several minutes capturing the unincinerated moths in his cupped hands and carrying them gently to safety outside. Before that, six raccoons lined up as he sat on a log, doling out snacks.

Ward had several field guides; from his animated and accurate descriptions of wild plants and birds, I knew he had read them.

Though he served in a very tough war, Ward opposed violence of any kind, including violence in nature. When our conversation turned to predation, he surprised me with the comment, "That's one place where I have a quarrel with the Lord. There should be no need for stronger animals killing weaker ones."

"But," I protested, "that is nature's way of population control to assure that prey species do not exceed their food supply." I should have known that was a poor choice of terms to use with a Catholic priest!

"Nonsense. No matter how rapidly a population grows, God's power of creation is infinite and He could create an infinite number of planets, even galaxies, to care for all the organisms that could ever reproduce and need space and food."

When my arguments failed to persuade this man of the cloth, I snorted, "That's the damnedest rationale I've ever heard. Let's call it a night."

"Sounds good. But first, let's have a nightcap and go for a walk. I want to show you how foolish bureaucracy can be." So, with port and brandy in hand, we began an outhouse tour.

"California Department of Parks is going to remodel all the restrooms. I'll show you a remodeled one."

Ward was right. There were no hooks for hanging up clothes or towels when you shower. You had to reach across and under the showerhead to turn on the water. I tried and received a blast of cold water in my ear. Tiny washbasins had faucets so far down in the basin that I bruised the backs of my hands trying to wash next morning.

An old restroom in the campground where I had showered last night was comfortable, convenient, much nicer—but slated for "upgrading."

Agreeing on restrooms and bureaucratic absurdity but not on predation, Ward and I toasted each other in the middle of the campground at midnight and went our separate ways.

ᗡᗣ ᗡᗣ ᗡᗣ

Sloshing northward through rainsquall after rainsquall, I thought about my days in the redwoods. Since first encountering redwood forests near Healdsburg, I had pedaled 304 miles to Crescent City before detouring to nearby Jedediah Smith Redwood State Park. There, I spent a day hiking and photographing in this moist, deep forest that also included Douglas fir, lodgepole pine, and knobcone pine before leaving the stately redwoods behind.

Three hundred and four miles of contrasts. Scenes of mystical beauty and haughty grandeur that evoked feelings of pride in America. But much had been lost—forever. I read that in 1921, the year I was born, there were 2 million acres of redwood forests. Now, after sixty-five years of logging and other uses, there were only about 300,000 acres of virgin redwoods remaining.

Properly performed, logging is a useful tool in forest management. But, as the California Coastal Commission had aptly pointed out, "Excessive and often poorly managed logging prompted the establishment of park lands to preserve some of the most scenic redwood forests."

Having grown up in logging and sawmill communities and worked briefly as a lumberjack, I truly understood that some of these activities whereby our hardworking forebears wresting a living from an unyielding land. But much destruction was done by exploiters seeking to wrest the bottom dollar from these irreplaceable treasures—regardless of consequences. One consequence was that some, who hadn't participated in the profits, now lived in conditions of environmental squalor.

The battle to further diminish these rich resources will continue. I only hope that the American people have the will to insist that society resists temptation for short-term profits in favor of enduring stewardship of the land.

I crossed into Oregon in a downpour.

CHAPTER EIGHT

Pacific Northwest

The mountains of the Pacific Northwest are tangled, wild, remote ... Here man can find deep solitude, and under conditions of grandeur that are so startling he can come to know both himself and God.

—William O. Douglas,
Of Men and Mountains

"I hope you took out a life insurance policy before leaving home," boomed a big lumberjack in Gayle's Other Place, where I stopped for breakfast in Brookings, Oregon. He and three other loggers warned me of narrow, winding, hilly roads jam-packed with logging trucks. Positive thoughts for a new day!

Oregon is known for having the toughest environmental and land-use laws in the nation. In the 1970s, popular governor Tom McCall reflected majority view when he told a group of conventioneers, "Welcome to Oregon. While you're here, I want you to enjoy yourselves. Travel, visit, drink in the great beauty of our state. But for God's sake, don't move here."

The first few miles into Oregon were quiet, almost mystical, as light drizzle splattered my glasses and my bike tires squished softly on wet pavement. It was so pleasant I amused myself by visualizing Gene Kelly dancing to "Singing in the Rain." As the rain slackened then stopped, shafts of sunlight illuminated billowing ocean fog. Fog banks lifted, revealing sailboats with bows splitting the waves as they tacked north into the wind. Between the highway and low cliffs ran an undulating ribbon of grass. Three ewes with their lambs pretended I was chasing them as they ran alongside for nearly a mile.

The white sheep, wet emerald green grass, and white-sailed sloops and ketches on the blue Pacific exuded old-world charm, bringing a peace that penetrated my being.

Near the top of a steep hill south of Port Orford, a station wagon eased past, pulled off the highway at the summit, and waited for me to catch up.

"Know what your expression reminded me of when I passed you and again just now?"

"I give up. What?"

"The little locomotive chugging up a grade while saying 'I think I can, I think I can.' Near the top, you had a big grin that said, 'I know I can, I know I can!' You look like a guy who enjoys what he's doing."

Rich Armstrong, an interesting and enthusiastic man, showed he was also impulsive when he said, "I have a cabin on the Rogue River where I conduct whitewater rafting in the summer. I'd like to have you be my guest on one of those trips. But first things first: I live on Saunders Lake seventy-five miles north of here. You should be there by tomorrow night and you are invited to stay overnight so we can visit."

The next day, I pulled off U.S. 101 eight miles north of North Bend and followed a winding road to Saunders Lake where Rich greeted me. He taught earth science and geology at North Bend High School; he also coached baseball and supervised the weight-lifting program. I discovered that Debbie Armstrong, an Olympic downhill ski champion, was his niece.

After I unloaded my bike and rehydrated with a beer, Rich suggested a hike over nearby sand dunes, described in a brochure as "dynamic yet peaceful." It was a quiet evening on the dunes and I agreed it was peaceful. But deeply gouged tire tracks, plastic food and drink containers, empty beer cartons, and other debris weren't my idea of "dynamic."

The brochure invited, "Come ... roar over the Dunes in an off-road vehicle." I expressed intolerance for all-terrain vehicles—ATVs—in areas of such beauty and potential quiet. Rich agreed. In the evening, he showed slides of the most spectacular sunrises and sunsets I had ever seen. Storm-whipped waves captured on film along the Oregon coast were higher and wilder than I could imagine.

⌬ ⌬ ⌬

After two days riding in fog and rain, I had discovered anew the difference between water-resistant and waterproof clothing, and I looked forward to visiting my cousin near Depoe Bay. The only thing Gortex resisted was the escape of steam from my sweating body. So I peeled down to T-shirt and biking shorts to ride the last dozen miles to Mary Ellen's beach house in cold rain and wind. Her husband, Ed, had explained where the key was located and instructed me to make myself at home.

An hour after letting myself in, I had a fire roaring in the fireplace. My bike, tent, and gear drip-dried in the shop. A load of laundry churned in the washing machine. Hot tea was ready to wash down homemade cookies that Mary Ellen had left when she and Ed had driven out the previous weekend from their home in Beaverton. Ed was an engineer with the Oregon Department of Environmental Quality and Mary Ellen had taught second and third grades in a private school for many years.

This was not the first time Ed and Mary Ellen had offered refuge. Shortly after Carol's funeral, they had recognized my need for solitude and invited me to spend time here in their beach house. I would run each morning, spend hours reflecting and walking on the beach, and write letters to people who had been kind and supportive during Carol's illness and death.

Now, at Ed and Mary Ellen's house again, I faced the Pacific over a card table loaded with mail picked up in Newport. Wind-driven rain swept across the windows, the foaming surf crashed against the rocks below, and a fire crackled in the fireplace. By nightfall I had read all my mail and written fourteen letters.

After three days of rain, Saturday morning dawned clear. Ed and Mary Ellen drove out for the weekend, so I rented a plane and took Ed for a flight along the coastline. Viewed from above, the landscape unfolded in panoramic detail. A few days before I had biked along coast-hugging U.S. 101, but had not seen starkly beautiful Heceta Head Lighthouse a few hundred yards away, nor had I been aware that sea lions were barking and basking in a rocky cove a hundred feet below my spinning wheels. Swooping low to photograph this coastal community, I now felt more connected to land, ocean, and sky.

In *Chasing the Glory: Travels Across America,* Michael Parfit described following Charles Lindberg's footsteps in the sky. In 1928, the year after flying a small plane alone across the Atlantic, Lindberg flew 22,000 miles while touring the United States to promote aviation. Nearly sixty years later, Parfit repeated the feat by flying into all of the lower forty-eight states, landing at the same eighty cities where Lindberg had visited. Parfit wrote:

> *I have never known a land until I have flown with it. I don't mean arching high above in a jet. I mean ducking through the passes in its mountains; bounding on the humps of warm air thrown up by its fields. Flight close to the land gives you both the big view and the detail, and shows you how they connect.*

A spouting whale caught Ed's eye. I banked westward for a closer look. Excited by the sharp image of the whale in the clear water below, I inched seaward in search of other whales until Ed remarked that I had no training in ditching a plane at sea and no aquatic survival gear aboard. He wondered if we were getting too far out to glide back to land if the engine failed. He was right. I turned landward immediately, realizing that enthusiasm can kill if it obscures good judgment.

I resolved, though, to find more opportunities to add this aerial dimension to my view of America.

As I rolled northward, the sign "Tillamook" and a nearby herd of Guernsey cattle grazing in a lush pasture reminded me that in 1931 I had scraped together five dollars and purchased a heifer calf from a Tillamook dairy farmer for my 4-H Club project. At that time this region of Oregon was already famous for its outstanding Guernseys.

Fifty-four years later, I now followed signs leading to the Tillamook Cheese Factory, where I sampled enough cheese to suffice for lunch. Back on my bike, I squished for miles on wet highway and endured sloshing after sloshing of muddy water from passing vehicles. Finally, I checked into City Center Motel in Seaside to take stock and regroup. Steam rose from my body as I took off wet clothes, soaked from the outside by rain and the inside by sweat. Rain had relentlessly challenged my resolve for three consecutive days. Grateful for garbage bags, I opened one and pulled out dry sweatpants and shirt to wear to the Laundromat and later, to Hara's Restaurant for a superb seafood dinner.

An old-fashioned mass the next morning served up religion fast-food style. The priest delivered a dull, impersonal homily and got us out of there in twenty-nine minutes flat. As always, though, I felt uplifted after receiving communion with my Christian brothers and sisters.

After mass, I stopped at the Mug for breakfast. A young cyclist came in and I invited him to join me. Dave Kehmeier was riding from his home in Seattle to San Francisco. The previous year, after graduating in mechanical engineering from the University of Colorado, he had bicycled for two months in Europe.

"My two cousins, Ken and Kaye, live in Colorado," Dave announced. "Know either one?" That was a long shot but on target. Ken had taken my class in ecology at Colorado State University a few years before. Kaye had reviewed my book, *Above Timberline,* for the Colorado Mountain Club magazine.

Seaside, once a bustling town, now was supported largely by fishing and logging. When overfishing and pollution reduced fish populations and over-harvesting of trees reduced timber supplies, the town turned to tourist demands for resorts and tacky gift and souvenir shops.

In *Exploring the Oregon Coast,* William Mainwaring wrote, "Seaside boasts the state's most popular beach, one so busy during the summer season that it has the Oregon coast's only lifeguard tower."

Despite Seaside's commercialization, I experienced heartwarming small town friendliness there. Early Monday morning, I took my muddy bike to the Prom Bicycle Shop for major cleaning and adjustments and paid for it with my Visa card. At another store, I discovered my Visa card was missing and called the bike shop but they were closed. I called my motel to ask if I'd left my card at the desk. "No, but the bike shop owner called. He has your card," the clerk reported.

"How did he know I was at City Center Motel?" I asked.

"He didn't. We were the fifth motel he had called to ask if a gray-bearded bicyclist was there."

The shop owner hadn't left his name, so I called the police for help in locating him. They knew the owner but he had an unlisted home number the police couldn't reveal. They called him, then got back to me, saying the owner was on his way to the motel with my Visa card. Throughout all this, the police were understanding, even apologetic for my inconvenience when they couldn't reveal the unlisted number. Thanks were all the bike shop owner would accept for his huge efforts on my behalf.

After two days in Seaside, I rode to Fort Clatsop, where the Lewis and Clark expedition had wintered in 1805 and 1806. A rare pileated woodpecker and I arrived at the fort at nearly the same time, and we were greeted by park ranger Dan Dattilio and others with binoculars. Of course, they were interested in the woodpecker, not me.

The Lewis and Clark expedition, after crossing the Continental Divide, had camped on the Clearwater River in Idaho while building canoes for the remainder of their journey. After floating 600 miles down the Clearwater, Snake, and Columbia Rivers, they first saw the Pacific in late November 1805.

On December 8, 1805, the expedition members began building Fort Clatsop, named after a friendly local Indian tribe. I was surprised that the log stockade was only fifty feet square. It contained five tiny cabins, three on one side, two on the other. Between these two rows was the parade ground. Ah, the military!

One cabin housed Meriwether Lewis and William Clark, who spent much of the winter working on their maps and journals. Next to the captains' quarters, interpreter Toussaint Charbonneau, his young Shoshone wife, Sacagawea, and their baby, Jean Baptiste, occupied a small cabin.

Captain Clark reported cold rain every day except twelve of the one hundred eight days at the fort. The hunters, however, kept them well supplied with meat and pelts for clothing and bedding. They killed one hundred thirty-one elk, twenty deer, and a number of beaver, otter, and raccoon during a three-month period. A three-man crew spent more than two months boiling seawater in large kettles to provide salt for use during the winter. The surplus, about three bushels, was packed and carried eastward when the expedition left Fort Clatsop on March 23.

Now, on April 29, 1985, the warm sun caused steam to rise from damp wood chips blanketing the path I walked to see a dugout canoe like those the expeditioners had hewn during that long-ago winter. Suddenly, a weasel dragged a recently killed cottontail down the path. To see what would happen, I charged the weasel until it dropped its prey and hid among the shrubs along the trail. Fifteen feet from the cottontail, I waited until the weasel hesitantly returned to grab its lunch; then it scurried down the path with me in hot pursuit. After repeating this sequence four times, I stood almost astraddle the cottontail while the hungry weasel repeatedly darted back, edging closer each time. Finally, in utter panic, it snatched its prey inches from my toe and scampered around a bend in the path. Guilt finally prompted me to stop.

My thoughts turned to the gentle priest, Ward Bowling, back in California at Prairie Creek park where he saved moths from incineration in his candles' flames and where he fed visiting raccoons. I was glad Ward didn't see me tormenting this poor little guy. Then I wished he could have witnessed this event. It might have convinced Ward that this predator was only fulfilling its ecological mission, thereby helping to delay the inevitable population crash of this highly cyclic prey species. On second thought, probably not. The priest, I fondly recalled, was a lovable but stubborn old codger.

▲ ▲ ▲

Facing a stiff wind out of the north, I crossed the Columbia River on the narrow 4.2-mile Astoria Bridge and was in Washington, the Evergreen State. Twelve miles north of Raymond, I missed a photograph of two black-tailed deer that trotted across the highway and disappeared into a clump of Sitka spruce. I was muttering to my tape recorder when a young man with long tangled hair and beard biked past, then stopped. "Thought you were talking to yourself, communing with nature or something," Ned Oliver grinned.

Ned had lived in Denmark for several years. While there he bought a frame, scavenged or bought components, and created the strange-looking bike he was riding. Recently, Ned had been biking in Mexico. "Where are you heading?" I asked.

"North in general. Nowhere in particular. When I run out of money, I'll hitchhike back to my home state of Massachusetts, find a job, and earn enough to pay for more bicycling."

"What did you do in Massachusetts?"

"Went to school mostly. Got a business degree from a small college near Boston, but the business world didn't appeal to me so I bummed around and finally wound up in Denmark. Took some teaching courses, became restless and quit before earning a teaching certificate. I did odd jobs and a bit of carpentry whenever the money ran out. Since the biking bug bit me, I haven't stopped turning the pedals for very long at a time. Speaking of which, I'll be seeing you," Ned called as he swung his leg over the battered frame and pedaled north.

Twenty miles later I caught Ned in Montesano where we had coffee and sandwiches in the Beehive Restaurant. This time we talked about his future. In his travels, Ned had become interested in nature. "What kind of training would I need to get a good job with the Forest Service?" he asked.

When I started talking about physics, chemistry, advanced math, statistics, and dendrology, Ned's eyes glazed over. "Well, I'll be seeing you," he promised again as he burned rubber to get out of earshot.

"You know, this is getting to be a tortoise and hare routine," I laughed as I caught Ned again ten miles up the highway in Elma. I envied Ned's free spirit and lifestyle, and wished I'd undertaken such an adventure at his age. But how many people in their sixties enjoy even a modest adventure like mine?

That evening, I called Charlie Combs in Tacoma. Charlie and I had known each other in Colorado years ago. It was his cabin that Alan Landsburg Productions had rented for my headquarters while I filmed Colorado high country for their TV series in 1971.

"Good to hear that you've survived and are still pedaling," Charlie boomed. "Opal and I will pick you up in McCleary tomorrow and bring you home to stay as long as you can. Then we'll take you back to U.S. 101 at Shelton. That'll save you twenty miles of hilly biking." I smiled at his well-meaning offer. People often wanted to save me hard biking, not knowing my motivation. I could have "saved" hundreds of miles by now if I had accepted such offers.

After I had a good night's sleep on a comfortable bed and enjoyed Opal's huge breakfast next morning, Charlie brought me back to McCleary. "Okay," he grumbled, "you and your bike were leaning on that stump. I've returned you to the exact same spot where we picked you up yesterday." I guess that Charlie thought I was a little nuts.

🚲 🚲 🚲

Port Townsend was picturesque and clean. A huge billboard boasted: "National Cleanest City Achievement Award." After seeing the huge Victorian houses and turreted, gingerbread-bedecked inns, I wasn't surprised to find Port Townsend was settled by sea captains and merchants from New England. They, along with other citizens, raised enough cash in the 1880s to build a mile of track in response to Union Pacific's promise to finish a transcontinental railroad with Port Townsend the key railhead for sea-lanes to the Orient. Seven foreign governments built consulates along the unpaved streets. A boom was on. But it didn't last long. After the population peaked at 7,000 in 1891, expectations to become the premier port in the Northwest were crushed when the deal collapsed and Union Pacific never finished the railroad.

Boat building and a pulp and paper mill helped the struggling town survive. But heavy logging on the peninsula depleted the forests and sent the wood industry into a nosedive, a common occurrence throughout the Northwest. Tourism was now the principal support for the 6,100 residents. Many of the Victorian houses had been converted to bed-and-breakfast inns. An artist told me, "You wouldn't believe the amount of creative energy in this small town."

My thoughts turned to the museums and art galleries I had visited between San Francisco and the Olympic Peninsula. Their paintings embodied remarkable insights into coastal landscapes. I wondered if those artists revealed more convincing evidence of environmental degradation than scholarly but dull reports written by foresters, ecologists, and other scientists.

George Catlin's paintings in the 1850s and '60s came to mind. His *A Whale Ashore—Klahoquat* portrayed a lonely, damply lush geography that foretold the ultimate fate of wilderness in an emerging industrial and land-hungry era.

Emily Inez Denny's untitled painting of Smith Cove in the 1880s vividly depicted the fantastic rate at which sawmills and stump-studded hillsides already had replaced nature's solitude and grandeur.

Between 1935 and 1943, the paintbrush of Morris Graves, who lived within view of clear-cuts, described what happened when a mountain was indiscriminately logged and its drainages were turned into gigantic mudslides. His art was titled *Logged Mountains*.

From the redwoods in California to the cedars, spruces, firs, and other conifers of the Olympic Peninsula, I saw only a few tiny remnants of pristine wilderness. A disturbing new landscape had emerged in the last few decades—a landscape of large, ragged clear-cuts featuring slash, stumps, skid roads, and eroded soil. Clear-cuts often became monotonous single-species stands planted by timber companies for maximum commercial values rather than for ecological integrity. Reminders of ravaged soil, forest, and mineral resources were the sad declining communities along my route.

Mulling these thoughts, I took a ferry from Port Townsend to Whidbey Island, rode the length of the island, then boarded another ferry to Mukilteo, south of Everett on the mainland side of Puget Sound. Riding north out of

Everett, I turned right on U.S. 2 and recorded, "This is it. I'm finally heading home!" The rugged crest of the Cascades was visible in the distance.

After fifteen miles of pleasant riding I was ready for breakfast at Petosa's Restaurant in Monroe, "Home of Washington State Penitentiary." Ten miles east of Monroe, I stopped at a general store to buy energy foods and film. My downfall came when the pretty girl at the check stand said, "From those muscular, tan legs I'd guess you were a bicyclist." Such flattery impelled me to invite her to come out and look at my loaded bike. As we talked, an elderly fellow drove up and unloaded newspapers into the stands in front of the store.

"Where you headed?" he asked.

"I hope to make Skykomish before dark," I called while swinging onto the bike and heading for the highway. Five minutes later, my "muscular, tan legs" were responding to hormones and flattery by driving the bike fast when I heard insistent beeping as a car pulled alongside. It was the man who had delivered newspapers at the store.

"Thought you were riding up to Skykomish," he shouted.

"Sure am."

"Well, it's behind you. I saw you pull onto the highway and head back toward Everett so I caught up to ask if you were lost."

I looked over my shoulder and there, clearly visible, were the snowcapped Cascades. With a silly grin, I thanked the old fellow profusely. Boy, a woman's flattery sure gets a man into a peck of trouble!

In Startup, I stopped at what appeared to be a church but was "Sky Valley Collective." The thirty-nine-year-old owner, Bill Miller, also repaired and sold parts for bicycles. Bill and his wife had traveled extensively on a tandem bicycle for Schwinn Bicycles. Bill, an exercise physiologist, had also worked with several exercise and cardiac rehabilitation programs.

After living in California, Shenandoah Valley of West Virginia, and other places, they kept drifting back to coastal Washington state, where they spotted this old church in Startup. Liking it here, they had bought the church and converted it into a bicycle repair shop four years before. They had a few antiques and what Bill described as "old stuff we needed to get rid of." Thus, Sky Valley Collective was born.

A few years before, Bill had bought a twenty-five-acre tree farm a few miles up the road from Sky Valley Collective. It was an outlet for his excess energy and restless spirit, and provided a little extra cash. A latent interest in trout farming led Bill to work a year for a trout farmer, and when we met, he felt ready to launch this new venture on his farm.

⚄ ⚄ ⚄

After ordering dinner at Cascadia Hotel in Skykomish, I quietly taped the day's events, ignoring glances from curious diners. Then, with a solid meat-and-potato dinner in front of me, I eavesdropped on three men in their thirties at an adjacent table. They were with a highway crew. Although their conversation was sprinkled with profanity, they impressed me with their thoughtful talk.

Next morning the hotel cook awakened me at 4:30 A.M. as promised. Coffee was ready at five o'clock and I was the first to order breakfast. It was still dark as early customers came in with reports that it had snowed all night on Stevens Pass. When it was light enough to see, I walked outside to find that cold rain was coming down.

As I drank coffee and waited to see how the morning developed, three burly fellows wearing suspenders and work clothes walked in. They were drillers with the highway construction outfit and would be going up toward the pass to prepare for blasting. In their late forties or early fifties, they were as quietly poised as the workers I had encountered the night before. Though robust cuss words punctuated conversation, there weren't the obscenities I had heard so monotonously and mindlessly mouthed by many university students in the late 1960s and early 1970s.

I put on rain gear and explored the village on foot. Skykomish is three blocks long, one to two blocks wide, and bisected by the railroad that comes up the narrow valley. Earlier, the waitress had asked, "Did the trains rolling by all night disturb your sleep?" I hadn't heard a sound!

Next day was Sunday and I was ready to move on after two nights in Skykomish. Some motorcyclists came in. They said it was icy on Stevens Pass. I would miss mass and ride anyway. My spirit shouted "alleluia" to be on the road again.

Pedals turning at 6:05 A.M., I estimated a four-hour, 3,800-foot climb to the pass sixteen miles away. The bike's blinking, battery-powered taillight reflected off the cold, wet blanket of fog.

Fifty-nine minutes and 6.9 miles later it was still foggy and cold, but sweat was pouring down my face and chest. Discomfort dissipated with the morning fog, and I was enchanted by the loveliness of two-foot snowdrifts surrounded by garlands of gargantuan, bright yellow jack-in-the-pulpits emerging through tapered margins of the drifts. Suddenly, tiny shafts of morning light slanted down through the clouds in preparation for a new day. Pure white clouds floated in a sky unbelievably blue. Spruce, fir, cedar, and hemlock were freshly covered with glistening snow that was getting deeper as I climbed. God and I, just the two of us it seemed, celebrated together these wonders of creation. I had attended mass after all.

I was jubilant when I reached the 4,061-foot summit seven minutes ahead of schedule. "Thank you, God. We did it!"

Quickly chilled, I stayed on top long enough to be photographed by a friendly tourist and to visit briefly with three others before saying, "Gotta get off this pass. I'm freezing!"

Wenatchee River Valley was filled with surprises. Somehow, I thought the Wenatchee would be a sluggish, dull river. Here, it was beautiful, bordered by large ponderosa pines and Douglas firs and with many rapids. The roar of

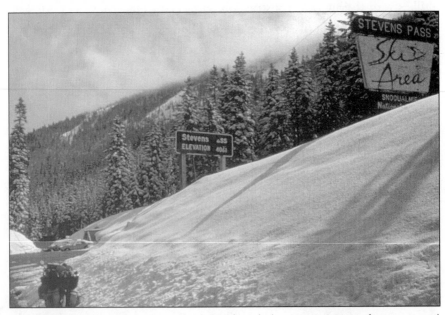

I celebrated completing the sixteen-mile, 3,800-foot climb to Stevens Pass in fog, snow, and cold; then interrupted questions from three tourists with, "Gotta get off this pass. I'm freezing!"

tumbling water tantalized me with my love for whitewater rafting. Spotting twelve climbers on a spectacular rock face four miles west of Leavenworth didn't arouse my envy, however. Except as a spectator, rock climbing is not for me.

Dollar-a-night bike campsites along the coast of California and modest charges at most other campgrounds had me spoiled. The eight-dollar charge at attractive Chalet Park in Leavenworth seemed high but turned out to be a bargain. After pitching my tent by a picnic table with umbrella, I leaned the bike under the umbrella for protection from heavy dew. The restroom was sparkling clean with an electric heater near the showers—the most pleasant shower I had experienced in dozens of campgrounds.

A tangy bratwurst and sauerkraut dinner topped off with apple strudel and a glass of rosé in Bavarian Village, a part of Leavenworth's business district, set the stage for a good night's sleep.

After burrowing into the sleeping bag, I gazed out the open tent flap to a dark sky spackled with millions of brilliant stars sharing space with fleecy white clouds. Once again, I rejoiced in the benefits of tent camping. Motel rooms often smelled of tobacco smoke, and the windows frequently wouldn't open. I seldom slept well and often awoke with a dull headache. Here, sleep came quickly.

The next morning, I was packing my tent when a man in a pickup pulling a huge trailer home tried unsuccessfully to maneuver into the park. I volunteered to guide him. After getting in without touching a thing, he thanked me profusely, saying he couldn't have made it on his own. I went back to breaking camp. A crash. Gushing water. Sparks. Profanity. He had gotten to his site with that monster, then backed it over a post supporting water pipe and power!

In freshly scented early dawn light, I pedaled out of the park. Despite four hills and light headwinds, I rolled 10.8 miles in forty-two minutes, a 15.5 mile-per-hour average. Pear trees were so loaded with lush blossoms I couldn't see the leaves. Apple blossoms were almost gone but still added a soft perfume to the air. What a contrast to the snow-packed Stevens Pass that I crossed yesterday!

In Cashmere I had breakfast and talked with four farmers, all six-foot-plus, more than 200 pounds, with big stomachs but solid as a rock. They said this community was supported by agriculture, mostly orchards. They mentioned communities on the coast that had gotten the big money. Then factories, mills, or mines had gone broke, often caused by changes in the markets.

"Those people hadn't learned to handle lower incomes," said Mr. Garrett, one of the farmers. "We've never had anything here anyway so we've learned to manage a good life without high incomes."

Mr. Garrett continued that he enjoyed more than 100 miles of cross-country ski trails in the nearby countryside. He also had a sixteen-foot sled-boat with a forty-horsepower outboard motor that was propelled by a jet of water ejected from the back. He could take the boat anywhere there was 1.5 inches of water and follow waterways fed by wastewater off agricultural lands in the Columbia River Irrigation Project. These waterways "go through country with herons, avocets, coyotes, and lots of nothing," he said, but Garrett liked it that way.

The three helicopters I had seen while coming into town, they told me, were used for spraying orchards, but more profitably for helicopter skiing in the winter and transporting hunters and anglers into the backcountry in season. Two of the farmers had experienced both kinds of recreation. I was sure these fellows couldn't appreciate the problems of living on five dollars an hour.

The conversation turned to Leavenworth, which I had described in such euphoric terms. The farmers called it a tourist trap that delighted business people who gleefully predicted a population increase to 12,000 in a few years from its present 1,500. Many folks, disliking the tourist orientation, went to Wenatchee to shop where more useful items were priced lower. The farmers agreed that local opinions were mixed but that most people liked to live in Leavenworth because it was an attractive town, had a good climate, and was close to a river and the mountains.

The well-maintained homes, neat lawns, clean and attractive business areas in towns, and the productive farms and orchards east of the Cascades were impressive. They indicated to me that these communities were more prideful and affluent than the logging, mining, and fishing communities I had encountered along the Oregon and Washington coast.

🚲 🚲 🚲

May 8, 1985. No exciting discoveries in the past twenty-four hours and sixty-two miles. No beautiful scenery. No scintillating conversations. Just sixty-two miles farther along; just sixty-two miles less to go.

At breakfast in Steamboat Rock Restaurant the next morning, three young fellows asked how many tires I'd worn out.

"Only one," I answered, "but I've had two flats from hitting broken beer bottles. Since the tires had quite a bit of wear, I replaced them at the next town." They expressed amazement at the amount of broken glass and trash I had encountered along the shoulders. Bicycling does sharpen one's recognition of people's trashy habits.

Later, over a cup of coffee at the tavern in Hartline, I spoke to the woman tending bar about all the empty beer cans and bottles I'd found along the side of the road. "Well," she said, "it's the open container law that is responsible. If they would just get them for drunk driving, it would be one thing. But when they stick them for open containers in the car, it's natural to throw their empties out to get rid of the evidence."

I suggested that people shouldn't drink and drive in the first place. "Well, I don't think drinking a few beers while driving is all that bad. It's the open container law that causes the problem." With that attitude, it's no wonder America's roadsides are cluttered with beer and liquor bottles and the police are kept busy making arrests for those driving under the influence.

🚲 🚲 🚲

In Spokane Father Ron Weissbeck, former pastor at my Fort Collins parish, John XXIII University Center, was completing graduate studies at Gonzaga University. He greeted me at the Jesuit House. My room was large and tastefully decorated. The bathroom had a big tub and huge shower. Water temperature could be adjusted exactly. I opted for 102 degrees and enjoyed a perfect shower. Toilet and lavatory were in a separate room. The bedroom had a large, comfortable bed plus a leather-covered ottoman, large desk, and dresser. There was also a television, which I didn't turn on. Floors were carpeted. Jesuits know how to live!

Ron and I walked around campus and saw the home where Bing Crosby was reared. It now houses the Crosby library. Then we strolled along the Spokane River and I could understand why Ron seemed so captivated by a city I remembered from the early 1930s as depressing, especially the dirty, junk-filled areas along the river.

We visited Riverfront Park with its opera house and convention center. Also in the park, we came upon forty life-size runners sculpted from wrought iron with an acetylene torch. From a distance, they looked like real flesh-and-blood runners. A bronze plaque honored the sculptor and donors: "The Joy of Running Together by David Govedare, 1985. A Gift to the City of Spokane by Individuals and Businesses in Friendship with the Lilac Bloomsday Association."

Asking about the remarkable renewal since the thirties, I found that civic leaders had long wanted to clean up the city. It took preparation for Expo '74 World's Fair to transform what was once skid row and railroad tracks into lovely Manito and Riverfront Parks along the Spokane River.

🚴 🚴 🚴

Signs informed me I had passed through State Line Village and was in my home state of Idaho. The next big sign proclaimed: "Andrea's Health Spa. Sexual Technique Analysis. Sauna Baths."

Somehow, the bold implications of Andrea's business fit the tackiness bordering I-290 much of the way from Spokane. This was not the highway I remembered from the 1930s when there were few cars, houses, or businesses— and certainly no traffic lights, which I now encountered at about half-mile intervals.

A few miles later, I visited briefly with my uncle and aunt, Loyd and Marguerite, in Coeur d'Alene. Soon my sister and brother-in-law, Leona and Roger, picked me up for the ninety-mile drive to their home in Moscow. Memories flooded my mind.

🚴 🚴 🚴

In the fall of 1939 I entered the University of Idaho in Moscow and studied agriculture until December 1941, when my studies were interrupted by World War II. Returning to the university in January 1946 and finishing my third year in agriculture, I then switched to forestry.

That summer I worked for a local contractor in Moscow who was building a small concrete block factory. After a thirteen-hour day hauling wet concrete in a wheelbarrow to pour foundations, I saw an ad listing a house for sale at $2,500. The price was right but I was too tired to look at the house that night. The next morning Carol and I found that it looked like a good buy but there was a "sold" sign in front. We were so eager to own a home, however, that I offered the new owner $2,750. After one day, he had turned a profit of $250 and we had a duplex with a one-bedroom unit downstairs and a one-bedroom unit upstairs, which we rented to a fellow student and his wife for $25 a month.

The contractor's next job, after finishing the concrete block factory, was to build a grain elevator a few miles north of Moscow at a site in the rolling hills of this easternmost extension of the Palouse, a large region in eastern Washington and northern Idaho lying north of the Clearwater and Snake Rivers. The Palouse, with its rich, deep topsoil, produces one of the highest nonirrigated wheat yields in the world. But there are values beyond economic. These wind-sculpted hills, vibrant green in spring, literally became "amber waves of grain" by late summer.

᚛ᚖ ᚛ᚖ ᚛ᚖ

After visits with my sister and her family on Saturday and mass at the University Catholic Church on Sunday, I was back in Coeur d'Alene on Monday, ready to head east again on I-90.

Beautiful Coeur d'Alene Lake was dotted with sailboats as I pedaled out of town. The pleasant scene summoned memories of our "Senior Sneak" day in 1938 when my high school class in Saint Maries, twelve miles up the Saint Joe River from the lake, chartered the *Seeweewana* cruise boat and spent the day sailing on the Saint Joe River and around Coeur d'Alene Lake. Then, I saw only one modest cabin in each of a few secluded coves. Now, there were hundreds of homes, some cottages but mostly large vacation homes or permanent residences, circling the lake everywhere I looked.

A highway department pickup stopped. "Just chuck your bike on the back. I'll take you to the top," the driver offered.

"No, thanks. I've pedaled 8,000 miles without a lift. I'm not going to cheat now."

"Okay," the driver said. "I didn't want to pass you up if you needed help on this mountain." Two miles later I read "4th of July Summit, 3,081 feet." An easy climb, a low summit. Folks tend to underestimate touring cyclists.

The sign read "Old Mission State Park." I looked south to a high knoll overlooking the Coeur d'Alene River and saw what I remembered as the old Cataldo Church. This, too, unlocked a trove of memories.

Times were tough when I graduated from Saint Maries High School. There was no money for college so I often worked as a lumberjack in nearby white-pine forests, still leaving time to plant, cultivate, and harvest fifteen acres of potatoes from the rich river bottom soil along the Saint Joe River. By the fall of 1939, I'd bankrolled enough money to pay room, board, tuition, and fees for the next two years at the University of Idaho.

Early that summer I bought a 1929 Model A Ford pickup for thirty-five dollars. It could haul ten 100-pound sacks of potatoes. A rubber-tired wagon became a four-wheel trailer that carried another fifteen sacks, a total of 2,500 pounds. The forty-horsepower Model A could barely pull a full load up some of the steep hills to the logging camps and mines where I sold the potatoes at $1.10 for a 100-pound sack.

My mother, a tiny woman who never learned to drive a car, insisted on accompanying me on these potato-delivering expeditions. One day, after delivering a load to the cookhouse for Sunshine Gold and Silver Mine near Kellogg, we noted the old Cataldo Church on our return to Saint Maries. I unhooked the trailer beside the road before driving across the mudflat to what is now Old Mission State Park. Halfway there the rear wheels began to spin. Mother promptly put her determined five-foot-two frame to the back of the mud-spewing pickup and we moved a little, then halted again. Leaving it in low gear and setting the hand throttle, I would jump out and push too. When a little traction was gained, I would dash madly alongside and jump in. It's a wonder the old Ford didn't wind up totally mired in the swamp.

Now, I turned the handlebars and rode the smooth blacktop entrance road across the flat, which didn't match the vast swamp of my recollections, and arrived at a parking lot near the simple but attractive visitor center. The park volunteer gave me brochures that provided facts I had never even wondered about while growing up nearby.

After visiting the old church and nearby parish house, I sat at a shaded picnic table and read: "They were a peaceful, proud, intelligent, attractive tribe of Indians who lived in teepees while searching for game, fish, berries, and roots along the shores of Coeur d'Alene Lake and the surrounding territory. Originally called the Schee-chu-umsh, they were renamed the Coeur d'Alene Indians, meaning, 'heart of the awl,' by French trappers who considered them shrewd bargainers."

The Coeur d'Alenes were a spiritual people. When they heard that a neighboring tribe had "medicine men" of great powers, they wanted this magic for themselves. They sent word that the "black robes," Catholic Jesuit priests, would be welcomed by their people. In 1842 Father DeSmet sent Father Point to establish Mission of the Sacred Heart twenty-eight miles south at Mission Point, a site where I later had fished and hunted without a clue or question about its rich history.

Father Ravalli joined the Coeur d'Alenes in the late 1840s and began designing the Cataldo mission. Born in Italy, Father Ravalli was an incredible man who combined artist, sculptor, and physician with preacher of the gospel.

Construction of the mission church was crude in most respects. Large pine logs for columns on the mission portico were hand-transported from adjacent forests across the mudflat by the Indians, as were eighteen- to thirty-six-inch-square timbers that weighed up to six tons. Walls, eighteen inches thick, were built from large logs latticed with saplings, woven with grass, then caked with mud. Floors were hand hewn and wooden pegged.

In spite of limitations, Father Ravalli attempted to duplicate the elegance of European cathedrals. For example, chandeliers copied in tin from used cans and crosses carved in pine adorned the interior. The main altar was hand-carved from wood and carefully painted and veined to resemble marble—a touch of Italy in the Idaho wilderness.

More than 300 Coeur d'Alene Indians worked on the project. An agriculture-based village emerged where, at any given time, at least forty people lived. Their idyllic life, however, was to be short lived. By the 1870s, they were feeling pressures from white settlers. In 1877, the U.S. government ordered them to move to a newly designated reservation sixty miles away. For a few years the Coeur d'Alenes passively resisted but finally gave in, left their special church and village, and moved south for a new beginning. There they built a new mission and eventually a school at a place named DeSmet after the old priest who had responded to their spiritual needs forty years earlier.

How sad that our government should severely disrupt the lives of a people who had labored so loyally to create a place of beauty in which to worship and to build a self-sustaining village where they raised their families.

ۼ ۼ ۼ

It was time to bike on to the home of Dr. Charles Hibbard and his wife, Colleen, in Wallace, Idaho. Chuck had been our optometrist in Salmon, Idaho, more than thirty years before and he had managed the nearby Lost Trail Ski Area where my two oldest children learned to ski. The Hibbards had invited me to stay overnight.

I found that Chuck was a program chairman without a program for that night's Rotary meeting. "Do you have any slides of your bike trip?" he asked. I admitted that I had picked up four boxes of just-developed slides at my sister's house but hadn't looked at them yet. "Good enough. You're our program for tonight." In forty-five minutes, I had washed up, put 144 slides in trays, and was enjoying a Rotary Club dinner.

It worked out okay with only a few slides that I couldn't identify. The Rotarians were appreciative and dinner was excellent.

🚲 🚲 🚲

I rode in light rain to 4,680-foot Lookout Pass on the Continental Divide and was in Montana. There were several truckers at Mary's Cafe in Saint Regis where I enjoyed noontime biscuits, gravy, bacon, eggs, orange juice, and coffee after a fast ride down the east slope of the Rockies. One trucker said, "Boy, you made good time coming down the canyon this morning. I passed you back about twelve miles."

Another chimed in, "Yeah, you were really smokin' when we went by." This praise reassured me that not all drivers of the big rigs hated cyclists!

The next morning I fought headwinds before meeting my former wildlife professor, Dr. Les Pengelly, at the Bill Johnson Airport near Missoula. It was too windy to fly as planned, so I rode to Les's home to clean my equipment, shower, rest, and visit with Les and his wife, Mary. The following day dawned clear and calm. I handled the airplane and Les operated my camera as we glided on smooth air over Frenchtown, Superior, Happy Hollow Ranch, the snow-capped Bitterroot Mountains, and the Diamond Match plant in the valley, before flying over sawmill smoke into Missoula's smog.

I thought of Lindberg's and Parfit's eloquent praise of small planes for understanding the landscape. I had taken the better part of two days to travel a hundred miles from the Continental Divide along the Saint Regis and Clark Fork Rivers to Missoula. Often battling headwinds, I had seen little except the highway and glimpses within the narrow confines of the mountain valleys; but during my 1.4-hour flight with Les, the mountains, valleys, villages, tiny pastures, and forests came together in patterns that made geographical and land-use sense.

Reluctantly, I left the Pengellys' hospitality and quite by chance, found myself riding with 617 Tour of the Swan River Valley bicycle riders who would ride 220 miles in two days. Their pace was faster than I'd been riding. But, riding hard, I managed to stay with them for eight miles until they turned north on Highway 200. Continuing eastward on I-90, I felt invigorated. It was time to pick up the pace a bit. I had been loafing.

I turned off I-90 at Garrison Junction to climb steeply along the Little Blackfoot River. Headwinds were heavy. It began raining. I covered the odometer with plastic.

The driver of a red hatchback beeped his horn, pulled in behind, and followed closely. I was a little nervous until he called out something about getting out of the rain. I stopped and a fiftyish balding fellow in a business suit stepped out and offered to tie my bicycle on the back of his car. Even if I wanted to, there was no way to tie this heavy bike on his hatchback. "No, thanks. It's not a bad storm. I'm doing fine."

I stopped at Avon Family Restaurant to gain energy for the last nine miles. After dinner a handsome young man and his wife at an adjacent table asked about my experiences. They both enjoyed bicycling but were sometimes upset by the attitude of drivers. As we walked out the door together, I commented that he must work out-of-doors since he had such a deep tan. "Yeah," he grinned, "I'm a logger." Fortunately, my complaints about logging truck drivers had been uncharacteristically gentle.

After riding 95.6 difficult miles, I registered at Last Chance Motel in Elliston at 9:15 P.M. It had been a long day.

The next morning the urge to move on was strong. I left at daybreak without breakfast. Six miles later a sign announced "MacDonald Pass, Elevation 6,325." I couldn't believe how easy it had been to climb to the summit on an empty stomach. From there, I would travel 480 miles down the Missouri River to Wolf Point, Montana, where I had begun this trek a year earlier.

CHAPTER NINE

Down the Missouri

... One of the most beatifully picteresque countries that I ever beheld, through the wide expanse of which, innumerable herds of living anamals are seen ... it's lofty and open forrests are the habitation of miriads of the feathered tribes who salute the passing traveler with ther wild and simple, yet sweet and cheerfull melody.

—**Captain Meriwether Lewis, writing of the Missouri River drainage not far from MacDonald Pass from** *The Journals of Lewis and Clark,* **edited by Bernard Devoto, retaining Lewis's creative spelling**

Astride my bicycle on the Continental Divide at 6,325-foot MacDonald Pass in Montana, I looked eastward. In my mind's eye I saw a molecule of water descending the eastern flank of the Rockies to the Missouri in which it would wander northeast, then turn southeast until joining the Mississippi at Saint Louis where the explorers' epic journey began on the May 14, 1804, and ended on the September 22, 1806. Ultimately this molecule, in theory at least, would flow into the Gulf of Mexico near New Orleans.

After these musings I took a long pull from my water bottle, left the pass, and let gravity provide a free ride as I headed east toward Helena. I stayed off the brakes and frequently topped thirty-five miles per hour, following U.S. 12 under canopies of lodgepole pine and Douglas fir. From time to time the road escaped

the trees to cross a grassy glade or meander down a tiny valley. Then the tran-
quility I was feeling was rudely interrupted. A sign read "Frontier Town." Behind
it stood statues of a buffalo, a grizzly bear on a turntable, and a dog on a wheel
affair that made him bob up and down. What profit motives fostered the building of these mechanical monstrosities in the midst of such natural beauty?

I thought back to earlier in the day when I was sweating up the last mile on
the west side of the mountain, enjoying the peaceful scene of dark forests scattered like carpets thrown carelessly over the rolling hills. Then, too, my serenity
had been trashed when I came to a pullout and found cartons of all sorts, pop
and beer cans, juice containers, and food-stained plastic and paper refuse from
fast food places. I counted ten empty oil cans. All this overflowed the pullout
and mingled with mountain flowers and blooming shrubs adjoining the site.

🚲 🚲 🚲

Helena, with a 1980 population of 24,000, was considered one of the
most remote and least populated state capitals in the United States. After
checking in at Super 8 Motel, I biked toward the Saint Helena Cathedral.
Black clouds were building up. Thunder and lightning increased. Suddenly I
was drenched. An open side door to the cathedral looked inviting. I rolled my
bike inside. After a few minutes of reflection and prayer, I walked outside to
see if it was still raining. It was. As I scanned the sky, a woman stopped her car
and ran into the church. I returned inside and found that her name was Irene
Roberts. After the usual get-acquainted pleasantries, she spoke of her six children and twenty-seven grandchildren, then explained changes she had witnessed at the Saint Helena Cathedral.

Renovation of Saint Helena, completed three years before, was patterned
after Saint Peter's Basilica in Rome. At one time, Irene said, they had the pulpit
high up in the front of the church. Later the pulpit was brought down to a
more central position and the railing removed so the priest would be more
among the people. This caused all sorts of dissension and arguments.

Irene and I agreed that some Catholics seem confused about the fundamental purpose and centrality of our religion: is it beauty and arrangement of
the church and form of the mass or is it people living their faith in service and
in love of God and community? We opted for the latter.

After breakfast next morning at the Country Kitchen, I biked to the Montana Historical Museum and State Library to learn more about this part of the country. Afterward, I rode to the Charlie Russell Museum and enjoyed the energy and hard-hitting realism in the paintings of Russell, my favorite western artist.

ᚼ᚜ ᚼ᚜ ᚼ᚜

I arrived at Lewis and Clark Landing on the Missouri River on May 19, 1985. Meriwether Lewis and his party had entered this same canyon on July 19, 1805. Based on Lewis's observations, it is now called "Gates of the Mountains."

Don Kurtz, a Landing employee, offered to take me down the river by canoe to Coulter Gulch. As we paddled downstream, it was hard to imagine that this canyon was once the floor of a great sea. The fossilized life vividly displayed on the limestone cliffs towering above us may be 300 million years old. Before the canyon's awesome grandeur and almost incomprehensible past, I felt infinitely small.

"I'll pick you up in the morning," Don called as he pushed away from shore and began paddling upstream.

After pitching my tent, I hiked a mile downriver to Meriwether Camp. From still-clear pictographs on the canyon walls, I tried to interpret stories told by Indians who traveled and hunted there 10,000 years ago.

Later, after crawling into my tent and snuggling into the sleeping bag, I left the tent flaps open to feel the brisk air, enjoy the stars, and listen to coyotes serenade the "honey moon," as they have for centuries. This full moon nearest the summer solstice has been known by many names, including the Indian name of "moon-when-buffalo-bulls-are-rutting." I felt invigorated, even if not like a rutting buffalo.

A cool river breeze ruffled my beard and hair, and I quickly fell asleep.

As early dawn light delicately suffused the tent, a cacophony of Canada goose, western grebe, and common merganser conversations echoed off the steep cliffs. I burrowed deeper into the sleeping bag, then heard songs that gently drew me to a waking state, sound by sound, moment by moment. First the sonorous sound of a mourning dove. Then a sprightly chirping, inflecting up then down in metronomic cadence. It was a robin's call, reminding me of reveille in the army. Time to be up and about. A rock wren joined the chorus with its remarkable repertoire of trilling lyrics. A western meadowlark urged me out of the sack with its loud flutelike melody. No doubt it was sitting, head cocked back, atop the stump I had noticed in back of my tent.

Thus, morning crept into my tent. As my friend Kevin Cook once wrote in his nature column about such a moment, "I listened myself awake. To immerse myself in the parade of life, I needed do nothing more than choose to notice."

Before breakfast I hiked upriver to Field's Gulch. An osprey slowly flapped its way upriver with me. Suddenly it plunged, legs outstretched, into the Missouri and emerged with a small fish wriggling in its talons.

A high-pitched, faint scream caused me to look up as I trudged back to camp. A red-tailed hawk soared above as it searched for breakfast, probably a fat ground squirrel.

After a night and morning close to nature, the blessed solitude was broken by the roar of an engine. Don had decided to pick me up by motorboat instead of canoe. We cruised down the river a few miles where Don hoped to find bighorn sheep. No luck. But we did see a mountain goat billy and nanny and their kid on a rock outcrop.

It was a varied and leisurely morning—a good break from the road. Back at the Landing I reluctantly loaded the bike for the steep climb to U.S. 15, where I started pedaling toward Great Falls.

Thirty miles later I noticed a bicycle leaned against a tree near a picnic table and restroom. Ready for a pit stop, I rode up quietly then inadvertently bumped my bike against the picnic table. A man, whom I hadn't seen sitting on the nearby creek bank, jumped up and spun around with a startled look on his face. He smiled weakly, "You scared the hell out of me. Thought you were a bear rummaging against the table. Name's Wayne Yankoff. Yours?"

That taken care of, we quickly got to important stuff—gear ratios, headwinds, close encounters with autos, and of course, miles pedaled daily. Wayne was training for a long bike trip. It was still morning but he had already ridden sixty-five miles and planned to ride a total of 120 miles that day.

I had been riding along, smugly recalling a recent 95.6-mile day, one of my best. I didn't suggest that we ride together.

🚲 🚲 🚲

At Holter Lake, I pitched my tent in a Bureau of Land Management campground, then rented a boat for a relaxing hour of rowing on the lake.

After a hamburger at Holter Lake Lodge, I returned to my tent to find a young man with long tangled hair, long unkempt beard, and his low-rider Harley standing nearby. A pistol butt hung from somewhere near his rear end. I decided to keep an eye on him.

Without introducing ourselves, we talked. He was waiting for his wife and two sons to come from town after the boys finished a Little League game. A big car drove up. His wife and two boys got out. Soon a campfire was roaring and they were cooking wieners. Things were quiet as I slid into my sleeping bag. Perhaps I had misjudged him.

Before dawn I heard a loud, high-pitched male voice and the Harley rider profanely discussing how they ought to bomb the bar and all the houses along that part of the lake to restore the area to its "wild condition." I chuckled, in the privacy of my sleeping bag of course, and concluded that they were harmless self-styled mountain men.

Later I stumbled sleepily toward the restroom. Walking past a huge husky tied near their camp, I reached down to pet him. With a savage roar, the dog lunged at me. I didn't move as he touched me with his wet nose but not his teeth. Lying on the ground, apparently awake and watching, the owner yelled, "My God, man! That dog is used to being in the mountains alone. You're lucky to still have your arm."

I still believe if you aren't afraid of a dog, they usually won't bite. However, not wanting to contribute "leg of man" for the dog's breakfast, I slowly, silently walked away without further testing this hypothesis. Reflecting later, I wondered if I really wasn't afraid or if I was half asleep and didn't know what the hell was going on. Anyway, it seemed a good time to strike camp and get out of there. I started riding at 5:47 A.M.

Two hours later a couple of white-tailed deer ran alongside. Every thirty steps or so they leaped high, their namesake tails waving proudly in the air. Soon, they left me behind. I passed them a half mile later as they swerved away from the road and disappeared over a ridge.

🚲 🚲 🚲

In Great Falls I began preparing for another weekend with Elisabeth. Checking in at Village Motor Inn, I soon busied myself washing biking gloves, shoes, helmet, and the helmet pads that helped fit the helmet comfortably on my head but absorbed so much sweat they soon became stained and foul. Then I aired out the tent, sleeping bag, and foam pad before going downtown to buy more film and film mailers, and to rent a car for the next four days.

Next morning, I checked out of Village Motor Inn and moved to a suite room in the Super 8 Motel. Now I was ready to drive to the airport to pick up Elisabeth.

Four days later, at eight in the morning, I returned to the motel after leaving Elisabeth at the airport for her early flight to East Lansing. Many feelings lingered in my heart. I needed time to think.

Quickly, I packed the bike and rode a few miles northeast of Helena to a spot that overlooked Hauser Lake. Hauser Dam forms the mid-reservoir of three that stub their toes against one another as they march down the Missouri River while impounding some sixty miles of the valley.

With a huge log as backrest, I sat facing the midmorning sun, reflecting on the four days Elisabeth and I had spent together. It had exceeded my fondest expectations. Hours discussing our possible future together flew by like minutes. Still, we found time to spend one day on a boat cruise through Gates of the Mountains with Jim and Addie Welsh.

Jim and Addie had been friends of mine in Fort Collins where they were members of John XXIII along with Carol and me. Jim, a colleague of mine, taught in the Agronomy Department at Colorado State University. Several years before, the Welshes had moved to Bozeman, Montana, so Jim could accept positions as dean of the College of Agriculture and director of the Montana Agricultural Experiment Station at Montana State University.

He had responded warmly to my letter requesting information about Montana and suggested we get together someplace "for old time's sake" when I pedaled through the state. Jim was visiting nearby Fort Assiniboine Experiment Station so meeting me at the Gates of the Mountains boat dock had worked out perfectly.

A few miles downstream, Jim, Addie, Elisabeth, and I had asked to be let off the boat. We would catch it a few hours later as it returned up the river. After a picnic lunch, we hiked to the site of the Mann Gulch Fire of 1949 that killed thirteen firefighters. Reading the plaque that described the fire and the deaths, I remembered

1941 when the Red Ives Fire burned thousands of acres of western white pine and other prime forest species in northern Idaho and western Montana.

I was working that summer as a lumberjack in a large logging camp in northern Idaho when our camp was called to help put out the fire. After we had been on the fire line a week, high winds brought flames roaring to the tops of 150-foot pines. This phenomenon, called "crowning out," causes even toughened lumberjacks to experience an adrenaline rush. Many of the firefighters were unemployed men hired off skid row in Spokane, Washington, for thirty-five cents an hour. They were terrified and began to mill around yelling, "Let's run for it."

Frank Johnson, boss of our logging camp, was near me. "Smitty, stay close and hang on to your Pulaski," Frank said before facing the panicked mob heading toward us on a narrow forest trail. "First man that tries to get past us gets a Pulaski in his goddamn face," bellowed the big Swede. The bluff worked because of Frank's imposing 300-pound frame, not because of the scared nineteen-year-old beside him.

A Pulaski is a tool with an axe on one side for chopping brush or trees and a hoelike tool on the other for digging down to organic soil when building a fire line. It was named for a legendary Polish firefighter who designed it after fighting the famous fire of 1910 that burned thousands of acres in northern Idaho and western Montana.

The crew prevailed, and we held our sector of the fire line that day. But a few days later we were caught with no place to escape except to follow a creek for a mile through recently burned and still hot countryside. We ran over blistering rocks and burning embers until our feet became so hot that we walked in the creek to cool them enough for us to run through the smoldering coals again. The next day the soles of my custom-made thirty-five-dollar White's disintegrated. Sixty years later, this famous logger boot sells for $325 and is still the favorite of wildland firefighters.

A year after this fire, I reported for work in a construction company that was building army barracks on a base near Kodiak, Alaska. To my amazement, the crew boss was Frank Johnson. I asked, "Frank, would you really have let them have it with that Pulaski?"

He grinned. "You'll never know. Neither did those guys." I think it was a bluff—but it worked!

🚲 🚲 🚲

After mass on Sunday, Elisabeth and I decided to drive to the mountains. When we reached Gibson Reservoir on the Sun River sixty miles west of Great Falls, I thought of a time in 1954 when Dr. Helmut "Hal" Buechner had hired me to assist him in a study of the Sun River bighorn herd as part of research included in his book, *Bighorn Sheep of North America*. He had been in the Gibson Reservoir area for some time but had not been able to approach the sheep closely.

Hal knew I had been studying the behavior of bighorn sheep in Idaho for four years and, on occasion, had gotten within ten or fifteen feet of the animals. He hoped I could get some close-up photographs. One day the sheep cooperated and I worked my way into a herd of fifty, including sixteen full-curl rams that milled around me. I photographed the magnificent animals until I ran out of film. No such luck this time. Elisabeth and I saw numerous pronghorn in the distance but no bighorns.

On Memorial Day we visited the Charles M. Russell Museum and the log studio where this famous western artist did much of his work until his death in 1926. Russell had worked as a cowboy and was a keen observer. He used the prairies he knew so well for his detailed paintings and sculptures that interpret America's frontier heritage with an integrity achieved by few other artists.

Later, we drove to Pishkun State Monument near Ulm. *Pishkun* is a Blackfoot word meaning "buffalo jump." On the prairie above a huge cliff, Indians hundreds of years ago built a broad funnel-shaped lane with sides of stones that guided buffalo to the precipice. Once herded into the mouth of the funnel, Indians hidden by terrain features and piles of brush alongside the lane would jump up and begin shouting, causing the buffalo to stampede. Animals in back pushed those in front over the edge. Indian men waiting below dispatched those not killed in the fall, and women quickly began butchering.

Reflections continued. During the four days Elisabeth shared with me in Great Falls, my emotions ranged from delight to guilt. Delight in planning a possible future together; guilt that the pain I often felt on quiet mornings and evenings as I revisited the pleasant landscape of my thirty-nine years with Carol seemed to fade with the flush of joy I experienced with Elisabeth.

漏 漏 漏

I found it hard to get started after leaving the motel and sweated profusely. After a few hours, however, the rhythm and cadence came back and I was rollin' again. Near the mouth of Maria's River, a historic site sign told that Lewis and Clark had camped near here for two weeks.

The *Journals of Lewis and Clark* capture, in colorful fashion, that Captain Lewis appreciated the beauty of the ladies and recognized the nobility of a pristine river. On June 19, 1805, he described how he named the river:

> *I determined to give it a name and in honour of Miss Maria Wood I called it Maria's River. it is true that the hue of the waters of this turbulent and troubled stream but illy comport with the pure celestial virtues and amiable qualifications of that lovely fair one; but on the other hand it is a noble river.*

🚲   🚲   🚲

Seven miles north of Loma, Jay Worrall was getting mail from his mailbox. "Where are you heading?" he called as I pedaled past. A half hour later I moved on with more appreciation of farming in this area, which Jim Welsh had described as one of the best grain-producing regions in Montana.

Buildings, fences, and fields of the Worrall ranch attested to a successful operation. Jay told me that two of his great uncles arrived in that country in 1912 and the Worrall family had farmed there since. With engaging modesty he said, "We've had lots of good luck." As an example, he said that in March 1981 huge crops of winter and spring wheat were forecast for this region, meaning low prices for wheat in the fall. Since they hadn't begun seeding, the Worralls seeded about 8,000 acres to barley. Yields and prices were exceptionally good that fall and had continued high. Jay concluded, "It's been a real windfall for us."

High yields and excellent condition of topsoil on Jay's land indicated that, rather than luck or "windfalls," it was love of the land and good farming practices that brought about the Worralls' success. I rode on, feeling good about Jay and his examples of "sustainable agriculture."

Still interested in land-use research, I called the Agricultural Experiment Station located at old Fort Assiniboine to see what was going on there. A researcher named Harold came to town to drive me to the station. A field day was underway at the station so the scientists, including Jim Welsh, were out in the pastures reviewing ongoing research. We drove out to join them. Many of the investigations were designed to determine optimum systems and intensities for cattle grazing on these grasslands. Their research techniques were similar to what I had used when I was a range scientist in charge of cattle grazing studies at a Forest Service experiment station in Colorado thirty years before.

Despite my nostalgic recollections of how we did research in the "good old days," I was impressed with the improvements in forage production and grazing practices that had resulted from research conducted at the Fort Assiniboine Station. For example, by planting alfalfa, vetches, and a variety of other legumes among nonnative grasses, they had increased forage production on dryland ranges from 200 pounds per acre to 1,000 to 2,000 pounds annually, which means they could produce five to ten times more beef. In Colorado studies with similar plantings, however, we found that production began declining quite rapidly after ten years or less. That result illustrated the difficulty of sustaining increased production by altering native grasslands.

If we continue to "over-people" our planet, however, such measures will undoubtedly continue and many, I predict, will fail in the long run.

With those apocalyptic thoughts, I realized it was raining heavily, the tour group was getting wet, and our drivers were wondering if they could get back to station headquarters over the muddy roads. They did, and we were rewarded with huge steaks grilled over charcoal, hot Boston-baked beans, cold potato salad, fluffy rolls saturated with butter, all topped off with a delicious home-baked cake. Happily stuffed, I was ready to return to Havre. Worries about breeding ourselves into oblivion would have to wait.

The next morning at 5:15 there were more immediate concerns. It was still pouring rain. I turned over and slept until 6:45, then listened to the weather forecast: Rain for the rest of the week. The morning paper reported that this area received an average of only ten inches of annual rainfall. Why was it all falling in June this year?

In spite of rain and a late start, I arrived at the Bonsoir Motel in Malta with 91.6 miles on the odometer before nightfall. After gracious permission from the manager, I spread newspapers over the floor and rolled my dripping bike into the room. Then, I removed the handlebar bag and four panniers, emptied them completely, and piled the contents on newspapers to let them dry.

After a shower and leisurely dinner, I wiped down Old Faithful, rolled her out to the parking lot, and began the ritual of oiling chain, gears, and other moving parts; then I took a couple of loops around the motel while running through all eighteen gear combinations to distribute the oil evenly.

At day's end I called Elisabeth. Her voice was so warm and filled with positive feelings that I charged enthusiastically into twenty minutes of stretching exercises. I was ready for bed at 11:30 P.M., knowing I'd sleep like a log.

After a good breakfast next morning, I felt even better about my call to Elisabeth. A banner day, indeed!

🚲 🚲 🚲

Three fiftyish ladies in the Hinsdale post office asked about my trip when I stopped to mail a tape cassette to Sandi. As I prepared to leave one smiled and said, "Well, have a good trip." Another remarked, not intending for me to hear, "Whatever it is you do this for." Many people seem to feel that the only valid reason for travel is to get from one place to another as quickly and comfortably as possible. They make absolutely no sense of the purpose, logic, or challenge of a trip like mine.

In Glasgow I stopped at a Dairy Queen for an ice cream cone. A woman across the street stopped her car and called out, "Didn't I see you about a year ago in Wolf Point with those yellow saddlebags?" Eleven and a half months before, I had, indeed, been heading east out of Wolf Point to begin this journey. She had a good memory.

At Nashua it became apparent I couldn't make it to Wolf Point before nightfall so I settled for eighty-six miles when I met Stubby in the Nashua Bar and he offered his trailer as sleeping quarters. Another chance for a 100-mile day down the tubes. After getting into Stubby's trailer, dry for a change, I heard the rain begin to hammer the metal roof and congratulated myself for good judgment in stopping.

Next morning a cheerful waitress in Nashua's Home Cafe served the best old-fashioned country sausage I'd had in years, and I was on my way early. Black clouds were building in the west. I hoped to beat the storm into Wolf Point.

I did, although black clouds followed me all the way to Wolf Point where I checked into the Sherman Motor Inn. Then I toyed with the idea of asking a friend in Fort Collins to fly the Cessna to Wolf Point. I could enjoy flying it back to Fort Collins and be home in five hours.

"Wait a minute," an inner voice argued, "you're feeling fit, the Black Hills country is beautiful. It's only an extra 800 miles to ride." That decided, I spent the evening in a familiar routine—clean and lubricate bike, launder clothes, and shower.

Early next morning I was ready to ride through the Black Hills back home to Colorado.

CHAPTER TEN

Through the Black Hills

A number of my fellow chiefs and I are interested in finding some sculpture [sic] who can carve a head of an Indian chief who was killed many years ago. [We] would like to have the white man know the red man has great heroes too.

—quoted from two letters written by Sioux chief Henry Standing Bear to sculptor Korczak Ziolkowski who began in 1947 to carve the Crazy Horse Memorial from a 600-foot-high mountain in the Black Hills of South Dakota. Ziolkowski died in 1982 but his family continues the project.

My first thought when I awoke in my motel room the morning after biking into Wolf Point was, "I'm headed home." Only 800 miles to go! Even with headwinds and rain, I could average fifty-seven miles a day and achieve my goal of being in Fort Collins on June 16, Carol's birthday.

First, though, I attended morning mass. Father Jim Burkmeir's homily centered on mystery—the mystery of a beautiful morning like this that we do not fully understand, the mystery of awakening in the morning to be with someone we love, and the gift of that love.

My prayers were in thanksgiving for the life of Carol, mother of our four children, for the happiness she gave to others and to me during our thirty-nine years together. I prayed for my children Gary and Sharon and their spouses, for my grandchildren, for the privilege of so many father-son experiences with Alan and Mark before their untimely deaths at ages eighteen and seventeen.

Rolling south on State Highway 13W in clean Montana air on a bright Sunday morning, I praised God for the beauty of creation.

◟◟◟   ◟◟◟   ◟◟◟

Vida, Montana. A post office, a few houses, Saint Anne's Catholic Church, Vida Baptist Church, a Conoco station with an "Out of Business" sign, and little else.

Eleven miles south of Vida a country cemetery attracted my attention. Five families were interred there, each buried in a small plot of native prairie grasses. I recalled a similar cemetery in western North Dakota I had visited a year earlier. It, too, was final resting place for five families, each with its own small plot of prairie.

I thought of Grandview Cemetery in Fort Collins, where my sons rest beside their mother.

Riding on, I explored my feelings about the tiny cemeteries and small white churches I'd passed while cycling across western prairies. These good lands and vast open spaces somehow brought forth pioneers who, despite immense hardships, built stable families and formed cohesive communities. Their heirs and successors seemed to share in pride of ownership. Tidy farm buildings and fields, well-tended lawns, shelterbelts, and windbreaks that were cultivated and clean gave evidence of lives well lived.

I suspected some people living here, particularly the young, might disagree with my idyllic perception of their lives. But it will be a significant loss to the nation if our economic and cultural structures evolve to a point where the family farm and this kind of life disappears.

◟◟◟   ◟◟◟   ◟◟◟

The Gladstone Hotel in Circle, Montana, was the kind of in-need-of-painting place I'd learned to avoid. When they said, "Your choice of any room for sixteen dollars," my skepticism increased. But what a delightful surprise. Inside, everything was clean and neat. Three throw rugs on my room's linoleum floor were freshly cleaned. The bed looked new, with an attractive bed-spread and firm mattress. Appealing artwork adorned the walls, complemented by drapes in tasteful pastel shades of yellow, pink, blue, and gray. A genuine leather overstuffed chair and nice desk and chair invited reading or writing.

The bathroom was plain but the rose and gray-tiled floor was sparkling clean. Instead of thin white towels often found in small-town motels, plush gold-colored towels were folded in attractive triangles. A full box of "styled" Kleenex rested on a convenient shelf. The soft toilet paper with floral design had the first sheet folded neatly into a triangle. Definitely not a typical ma-and-pa operation.

A couple in their sixties had owned the Gladstone from 1946 until 1967, then the "call of the land" had led them to return to farming for the next ten years. By 1977 the hotel had become badly run-down and the new owners were in debt, so this ambitious and community-spirited couple sold their farm and returned the hotel to a profitable, upgraded hostelry. When I arrived, they had just finished polishing the maple floor in the large lobby. Stunning!

☙ ☙ ☙

In Lindsey a woman bartender with hennaed hair served a cup of coffee and two dry donuts before settling onto a bar stool next to another chain-smoking woman. Both watched a game show, never taking their eyes off the tube. At a commercial the bartender glanced out the window and asked, "Where you ridin' that thing?"

I laid it on her, concluding with, "For the last seven miles, I averaged over twenty miles an hour!"

Her unenthusiastic response: "You was ridin' downhill."

I swallowed my coffee along with my pride and silently sulked out the door.

Eight miles and twenty-five minutes later, I recovered my enthusiasm: the highway was smooth, the weather balmy.

I toyed with the idea of making all 132 miles to Miles City in one day. But by early afternoon, the tailwind had shifted to a direct headwind. The hilly terrain kept my speed between five and eight miles per hour. The wind was hitting the bike with such force, control was nearly wrenched from me. My entire body was fatigued and my attitude gone to hell.

At 4:20 P.M. I heard a loud report. My rear tire had blown out, completely wrecking both tube and casing. Nothing to do but pull out my new tube and fold-up tire. When I had bought it, they told me an "emergency" tire was hard to mount. It was. That fact, plus gusting winds blowing sand in my eyes and the tire casing, turned a fifteen-minute task into a forty-minute ordeal. I pumped the tire three times before reaching Terry, where I pulled into General Terry Campground and pitched my tent.

What had started joyously had turned into a hard day of riding only 86.6 miles instead of the 132 I had thought possible.

While eating dinner, I looked out the restaurant window and saw a family closely inspecting my bike and its cargo. Concerned, I rushed outside and met Gary Ryti, his wife, Myrna, and their two teenage daughters. Gary and Myrna had been planning some cycling expeditions for that summer. Gary, vice president of State Bank of Terry, invited me to stop by the bank in the morning so he could help find a new bike tire and get a doctor's appointment for me. I had pulled a wood tick off my back a couple of weeks earlier. Now the spot was swollen and sore.

The next morning in the camp store, the clerk asked, "How'd you sleep in that little tent?" When I mentioned the wood tick bite and that every time I rolled over the pain awakened me, he said, "Pull up your shirt and let me have a look." After a brief examination he exclaimed, "Boy, that looks awful. You better see a doctor."

Two hours later at the hospital, the doctor came in and handed me a vial with a half-thimble "core" of infected material and the wood tick's head.

At State Bank, Gary made several calls and found that Coast-to-Coast in Miles City had the tire I needed. The fold-up tire had fair pressure so I foolishly drank coffee and visited with Gary instead of cleaning sand out of the casing and repairing the tube. Bad choice. I used the pump a half-dozen times to ride forty-six miles to Miles City where Kyle at Coast-to-Coast mounted a new bike tire, adjusted the brakes, and worked past closing time. "Only charge is for the tire and tube," he smiled. Along with "Thanks a million," I handed him an extra five-dollar bill that he refused before rushing home to dinner.

While eating breakfast next morning, I read the local paper. In his column conservative George Will extolled pioneer values and lamented their passing. I also was tempted to romanticize the lives of homesteaders and others who had lived here in those early years. But, while finishing breakfast, I recalled the histories from the late 1800s through the depression and World War II that were depicted on stone in the prairie cemeteries I had visited and in conversations with old-timers.

Their tales described unimaginable travail. Women became prematurely old from hard work under stark conditions and gave unattended birth to children who often lived only a few weeks or months. Some men, worn and broken in spirit by ceaseless labor and overwhelming family responsibility, turned to drink, committed suicide, or withdrew into dour solitude. Families lived far from medical services and stores where they could buy commodities that they couldn't make, grow, or raise—if they had any money. Access to what we now consider normal amenities was limited or nonexistent. Socializing consisted of family visits or functions at nearby country schools and churches. Knowledge of the outside world was limited to word-of-mouth, monthly journals, or perhaps weekly newspapers. Education often was limited to eighth grade—if they were lucky.

Farm families now had national and world news within the click of a remote control TV button and information accessible on computer networks, broadening their world and increasing their expectations astronomically. Most were within minutes of well-stocked shopping centers. On this trip I had seen ultramodern electronic and farm equipment not imaginable as recently as the booming 1950s. It was common to hear farm folks exchange stories of vacations to Alaska, Hawaii, the Bahamas, Europe, Asia, the Holy Lands—you name it.

I reflected that, though today's farmers and ranchers may not have to endure the deprivations or never-ending hard work of their forebearers, crops still must be planted, cultivated, irrigated, and sprayed during critical seasons. Timing is of the essence when crops are harvested. Around-the-clock attention may be needed during calving, lambing, foaling, or farrowing seasons to assure successful reproduction in cattle, sheep, horses, or hogs. Despite mechanization, there still is dirty, hard "stoop labor" involved.

A sign in a local restaurant read: "Don't cuss the farmer while your mouth is full." Good advice!

ᘓᕀᙓ   ᘓᕀᙓ   ᘓᕀᙓ

The twenty-one miles between "Howdy, You Are in Big Wyoming" and "Welcome to South Dakota" on U.S. 212 took me diagonally across the northeastern corner of Wyoming.

In the rolling country between the Little Missouri and Powder Rivers, a small airplane swooped overhead as I climbed to the crest of a hill a few miles north of Hammond, Montana. Later, I mentioned to the proprietor of the Hammond Cafe that the pilot seemed to be looking for a place to land.

"Yes," replied the lady, "a rancher just landed on the highway to pick up his mail. A lot of them fly in for mail at the post office next door, then come over here to eat and visit. We had a dozen planes the other day."

I told her that a state patrolman had once chewed me out for landing on a remote stretch of highway in Idaho. He said that having to land for a pit stop wasn't an adequate reason.

"Well," she replied, "I don't know about that excuse, but pilots here often have 'emergencies.' The gas gauge shows near empty, or they think they smell smoke, or the compass is acting up.

"Nobody bothers us anyway," she concluded, "and we use the highway as a landing strip all the time."

۞ ۞ ۞

I found a specialness about Spearfish, South Dakota, a town of 5,251 according to the 1980 census. At the combination service station, country store, sandwich shop, candy shop, and ice cream parlor, I headed for the ice cream parlor where, seeing the sweat coursing down my cheeks, the lady behind the counter brought two large glasses of ice water before taking my order. After creating a spectacular banana split, she told me that she and her husband had been in Spearfish for three years. Her husband had been in the National Park Service for many years where he served in Shenandoah Park in Virginia, Blue Ridge Parkway in North Carolina, Everglades in Florida, two national parks in California, and one in Arizona before coming to the Black Hills where he began working for the U.S. Forest Service. They loved the Black Hills and decided to buy this business. "Now," she stated emphatically, "we want to live the rest of our lives right here."

At the city park I pitched my tent beside a tumbling creek reported to be one of the cleanest in the United States.

Later, at the Brass Bull Restaurant, I met Dick Termes, internationally acclaimed artist, who had designed a system he called the "Termesphere" that displayed artwork on a large, revolving, lighted plastic ball. He had built several, given seminars on this type of art at Black Hills College in Spearfish, and was preparing for another seminar in Deadwood that evening. His friend Irv Crambeck took me out to see the creative and beautiful Termesphere on Dick's lawn.

We then toured the Black Hills College campus and the Passion Play site. This dramatic performance, one of Europe's oldest productions, is not what one would expect in a small town in South Dakota. Director and producer Josef Meier was born in Germany, became a U.S. citizen in 1938, and brought the Passion Play to Spearfish in 1939. It was no small undertaking. The huge stage faces a semicircle of seats. A fitting background for the open-air stage is colorful Lookout Mountain. The parking lot holds more than 1,000 automobiles.

Irv told me that many Black Hills residents are members of the professional American Stage that forms an ensemble of 250 players. A lighting system illuminates each scene with quality and quantity of light ranging from a moonlit night to early dawn, and from the bright glare of high noon to a multicolored Palestine sunset. Realism extends to releasing pigeons from cages as merchants and moneylenders are driven from the temple.

Civic pride was evident in Spearfish. Streets and sidewalks were clean. Neatly mowed lawns surrounded attractively painted homes and several geodetic domes. Irv said Black Hills College had talented instructors despite low salaries, and many creative and artistic people lived in the community.

Early the next morning, I entered Spearfish Canyon on a smooth highway with three-foot shoulders. I climbed at a steady pace, first through colorful stands of oak and other hardwoods, then through ponderosa pine forests. The forests and unique geological formations attract students in summer from Lehigh, Kent State, Penn State, and other universities to study natural resources.

Within ten miles of Spearfish, I passed Homestake Mining Company Hydroelectric Plants 1 and 2, each humming busily inside old-fashioned brick buildings surrounded by manicured lawns.

I spent so much time taking pictures, recording signs, and just enjoying the canyon that it was midmorning when I reached the much-recommended Latchstring Inn. Over a breakfast of coffee, three thick blueberry pancakes, and one trout, I scanned a booklet entitled "Latchstring Inn and the Conquest of Nature in Spearfish Canyon." The inn had begun modestly as a one-room log cabin in 1892. The sawmill and surrounding cabins were named Savoy. "Much of the canyon, until the coming of the railroad, was inaccessible to travelers as it was impossible for even a horse to penetrate the dense undergrowth," according to the booklet.

That was hard to imagine after my easy pedaling. Even harder to visualize was that the railroad was completed by hand, horse, and mule in 1893, described by an accountant with a penchant for detail as "31.91 miles of sheer up and down hill climbing through 375 curves, or a curve for every 436 feet." Air-conditioned and comfortable motorists, even hard-pedaling sweaty bicyclists, should appreciate the incredible efforts our sturdy forebearers put forth so we could travel this spectacular canyon so easily today.

Reluctant to leave the canyon, but feeling some discomfort from where the doctor in Terry, Montana, had removed the embedded wood tick head from my back, I stopped in midafternoon at Spearfish Canyon Lodge and rented "Wild Bill," a rustic cabin. Warren and Elinor from Saskatchewan took the cabin next door while I was doing my laundry. After examining Old Faithful with her travel-worn panniers, they invited me to go with them to Lead (pronounced "leed") for dinner.

At the Mother Lode Restaurant, we were told Lead's Homestake Mine produced more gold than any other gold mine in the Western Hemisphere. Some of its 200 miles of tunnels reached 8,000 feet underground. The waiter told us that Deadwood, just northeast of Lead, was where such colorful historic characters as Calamity Jane and Wild Bill Hickok were buried.

Warren had been in the art department at the University of Saskatchewan for twenty years. Elinor, a freelance writer, had taught writing and still wrote poetry. They each had two grown children. Warren had spent a year in Europe learning firsthand about European art and absorbing the culture. On another jaunt he took a three-month trek across Africa with a diverse group of people.

Our table talk was so animated we were startled when our waiter softly told us the restaurant was closing.

Next morning the traffic was light as I rolled quietly through a delightful mosaic of timber, grassland, and small communities. Most buildings were attractively designed to fit the environment. I recognized similarities between the Black Hills and parts of New England while "roller-coastering" the terrain and wending the curving highway that yielded scenic splendors around each turn.

At the Lake Pactola Visitor Center an informational sign helped me to understand the history of forest resources in this region:

The Black Hills National Forest is the first forest in the U.S. where timber harvest was regulated. More than 5,000 acres of trees were sold to the Homestake Mining Company on October 19, 1899. Logs were hauled to the sawmill by horse and oxen, sawed, then shipped by narrow gauge railroad to the town of Lead for use in Homestake Mining Operations. Sale No. 1 was signed by President William McKinley since authority had not yet been delegated to the Forest Service. This sale marked the beginning of forest management of public lands.

The Black Hills have supplied a young nation with a surfeit of natural resources. Many have been consumed or destroyed by ignorance and raw greed as well as necessary use. The untrained eye may not recognize that thousands of acres were once laid waste by logging, mining, road building, shoddy construction and quick abandonment of communities. Yet, as in other regions of abundant precipitation, remarkable recovery eventually occurred.

The lesson is, quite simply, that nature's wondrous powers of restoration have forgiven some of our past sins. But we must recognize that with continued abuse even the most resilient resources bend only so far, then finally break. Given some respite, and perhaps rehabilitative assistance, landscapes can return to captivating environments like Spearfish Canyon.

Many stops and two rolls of film later, I coasted downhill into the old mining town of Hill City. At the edge of town I noticed a large sedan waiting to enter the highway. When I was within thirty feet, the gray-haired lady driver and her gray-haired companion looked at me as she slowly pulled out. I squeezed the brakes and skidded sideways in sand while bellowing, "Dammit, lady, don't pull in front of a bike like that!" I felt silly as people at the corner service station looked up with big grins.

Geez! This was the third time a little old lady had nearly wiped me out. Nevertheless, I arrived safely at a Super 8 Motel feeling the day's rich experiences were ample justification for traveling only fifty-five miles.

The next day, drenched by a steady drizzle, I stopped at the bottom of the hill below Crazy Horse Memorial. The gateman thought I looked miserable and waived the dollar fee for cyclists. "It's a 35 percent climb to the memorial parking lot," he warned, "so you won't be able to ride up there with that heavy load anyway." Even reduced to my more realistic estimate of a 15 percent grade, I was proud to grind all the way to the top.

The mountain carving was obscured by clouds, but I dried out and had coffee and a delightful visit with sculptor Ziolkowski's widow, Ruth, and daughter, Monique. Both remembered "Dr. Ben," the noted neurosurgeon who had performed several surgeries on Korczak many years ago—the same Dr. Ben Whitcomb who had invited me to spend the night in his home in Maine last September.

In Edgemont, South Dakota, I bought a copy of the June 11, 1985, *Rapid City Journal* and was shocked to see, on the front page, a picture of Tom Sutherland with headlines that he had been kidnapped by gunmen in Beirut, Lebanon. Tom had been dean of agriculture at the American University of Beirut. A few years ago he and I had team-taught an ecology course at Colorado State University. Tom taught about genetics, his area of expertise, and I taught about energy flows, nutrient cycling, ecosystem characteristics, and related topics. Tom and I had lived three blocks apart and occasionally biked together to campus.

I was concerned about his wife, Jean, and their three teenage daughters, all in Beirut with Tom. It didn't seem possible. Tom was a brilliant free spirit, on occasion dressing in kilts and telling jokes in a broad Scottish brogue or breaking into a Scottish ballad—all to bring levity to an important point in his lecture.

The next day I needed to ride seventy miles to Lusk to assure getting home on June 16 as planned. Headwinds were substantial as I started riding at daybreak.

I was back in Wyoming again. After turning south on U.S. 85 at Mule Creek Junction, I was met by screaming headwinds. Nine miles and two hours later, I still battled the wind.

Twenty-five miles south of Torrington I stopped to admire and photograph the diverse landscape. A windmill pumped water into a tank for Herefords grazing the native grassland. Beyond the windmill a long, rocky escarpment formed by some ancient fracturing of the earth's crust dominated the horizon. Across the highway a strip-farmed field brought brief order to nature's wild abandon.

Walking back to the bicycle, I had one foot in the air when, right between my legs, a huge western rattlesnake "rattled." I jumped straight up three feet—more or less! The rattler didn't move. I dropped an abandoned tin can on its head. Not a twitch. Having spent years in rattler country, I wasn't tempted to poke it with my foot so I looked in vain for a stick. Returning to the spot marked by the tin can I found—nothing. At a faint sound, I whirled around. The rattler was behind me, coiled up, head swaying, fangs lashing out.

In years past I would have searched until finding a club or big rock, wished the snake happy rattling, and done him in. That day, with a grin, I realized how silly I looked hopping around to avoid the snake while searching for a "weapon." So, I took three photographs as it reared back and eyeballed me. Then, I left this piece of wild and wonderful Wyoming as I found it.

Leaving U.S. 85, I crossed muddy Bear Creek and even muddier Horse Creek before reading "LaGrange, Population 232." Most prominent of the few buildings in town was the Frontier School of the Bible.

After pitching my tent in the backyard of Jack Chamberlain, owner of the cafe, I walked to Frontier School to visit with Harold Grimm and Marsden Petersen, business manager and registrar. They quickly provided a school catalog and handout materials. The school had been established in 1967, "... in the will of God, it is believed He will maintain it both financially and spiritually." Apparently He has, because there were thirty-five students who were required to "subscribe to our doctrinal statement without reservations." This statement was summarized as: "We believe in the verbal, plenary inspiration of the Scriptures which in the original writings are inerrant, absolutely infallible and God-breathed. They are the supreme, final authority in all matters of faith and conduct."

I thought of my students and the times I had exhorted them, "Search for the truth even when it means questioning your texts or, heaven forbid, your professor." The best students sometimes took me seriously!

As a happily converted Catholic, I smiled at the description of cults, a required course in the senior year at Frontier.

A study of the history and doctrines of the major cults calling themselves "Christian." Emphasis is placed on Roman Catholicism, Jehovah's Witnesses, Mormonism, Seventh Day Adventism, Christian Science, and

Anglo-Israelism (Herbert W. Armstrong). Special emphasis is given to the use of the Scriptures in refuting the teachings of these cults.

I was appalled at the spiritual arrogance in implying that a two-credit course could give adequate background in the "history and doctrines" of six major groups of believers, let alone even a minimal base for "the use of scriptures in refuting their teachings." No wonder prejudices abound in our great land.

The ascent from LaGrange toward Cheyenne was gentle, the headwinds brutal. After two hours I calculated my average speed at 4.28 miles per hour and began steeling myself to meet the physical challenge of honoring my commitment to attend early mass in two days. The 115 miles to Fort Collins would be a piece of cake in normal conditions, but what is normal about Wyoming weather, I reflected somewhat bitterly as merciless winds buffeted Old Faithful and me. I promised aloud that I would make it to Cheyenne before nightfall come hell or high water.

After plenty of hell but no high water, I arrived at the Quality Inn near the north edge of Cheyenne at 7:05 P.M. It had taken more than twelve hours to pedal 56.1 miles. After a shower and dinner, I hit the sack, exhausted.

🚲 🚲 🚲

June 16, Carol's birthday. I rolled onto the highway at 3:11 A.M. By 5:33 I had finished breakfast at Little America, biked 15.3 miles, and photographed two signs: "Welcome to Colorful Colorado" and just beyond a bicycle sign and the words "Next 10 Miles Keep Far Right." It was good to be on I-25 in Colorado, and this was the first time I had seen legal status given a bicycle on an Interstate, although maps and brochures state that if there is no "reasonable alternative" and if bicycles are not "specifically prohibited," riders have the "same rights and responsibilities" as motorists.

I was feeling exuberant. The sun was just peeking over the horizon, and I was rolling at twenty miles per hour. Before this trip, I had seldom ridden that fast, even on an empty bike. It was great to be alive and good to be coming home right on schedule! I felt a bit wistful realizing I wouldn't be preparing tonight for tomorrow's ride.

What a change from yesterday. This morning I rode 55.2 miles, detoured to the airport to reserve a plane for tomorrow, stopped with friends for a cup of coffee, found the doors open at John XXIII University Parish, rode inside, and leaned my bike against the wall. By 8:10 A.M. I was in the small chapel, praying in thanksgiving for being blessed by the lives of Carol, Alan, and Mark, to whom this memorial ride is dedicated.

Later, I was seated next to the center aisle in the third pew from the front, a place Carol and I had occupied on Sundays for fourteen years. A friend came up and whispered, "Welcome home. We didn't know you were back until we saw the sign outside."

"What sign?" I asked.

"The one right beside the front entrance."

I walked outside. Sure enough, a large sign read, "Welcome Home, Dwight!" Totally focused, I had ridden within five feet of the sign without seeing it!

After 9,549 miles on the perimeter ride, it was good to be home.

ک ک ک

Before leaving Fort Collins at the start of my journey, I had rented my home to a Realtor and his family. Back again, I needed a place to stay. Not wanting to ask the renters to move, I rented half a duplex and set up housekeeping.

Bicycling became my main transportation in town. I renewed membership in my health club, began working out two or three times weekly, and ran four to six miles twice a week.

In the previous year I had flown only thirty hours, mostly to photograph or just enjoy the countryside from the air. Very little involved practice of rigorous maneuvers or procedures needed to maintain flying proficiency. Although a BFR (Biennial Flight Review) wasn't required for another eleven months, I needed flight training for safety's sake.

My original flight instructor flew with me one day and agreed I needed to brush up on landing technique as well as steep turns, stalls, spin recovery, and a few other skills that had accumulated rust. After several hours of instruction, I felt more confident and flew several cross-country flights solo or with friends.

ک ک ک

In August, Elisabeth invited me to join her high school class' fortieth anniversary celebration in Germany. We flew to Frankfurt, where we met Elisabeth's sister and brother-in-law, Karola and Willy, who drove us to their home. They lived in Mainz-Gonsenheim, a small town surrounded by rolling hills, scattered small fields, and forested areas. Most days I followed forest trails for an early run, visiting one or two villages before breakfast.

Each morning, Willy walked to a bakery and brought home a variety of fresh breads. These were served with an assortment of cheeses and slices of meat, including sausages. A pot of freshly brewed coffee was always ready.

On some days we rented bicycles and biked with Willy and Karola in the nearby countryside. We stopped at out-of-the-way family owned and operated cafes in small villages. The food and wines were superb. An all-day boat cruise brought memories for Elisabeth and appreciation for me of the beauty of the Rhine Valley, where vineyards and castles overlooked the river.

A daylong bus tour with Elisabeth's former classmates included a few World War II veterans who began asking about my war experiences. Initially I didn't feel comfortable discussing the campaigns in which I, as an infantryman, had fought against their troops. But their frankness and friendliness disarmed and amazed me. One insisted that after the war he was in a POW detail that reported to the section I had commanded. I didn't remember him.

The day before we flew back to the United States, he called to say he had a gift for me. He had selected books of photographs of the German countryside, pieces of artwork, and tasteful mementos. In heavily accented English, he confided, "I want you to know there were good people in Germany, too." He needn't have assured me.

ڶ ڶ ڶ

Back in Colorado autumn was approaching and it was time to begin preparing for the final segment of the perimeter trip. After a half-dozen fifty-to sixty-mile training rides, I boxed Old Faithful for the flight back to Charleston, South Carolina. Then I called the Crumps, who had opened their home to me in Charleston a year before.

Tim answered the phone. "Hey, Dwight. We've been expecting your call. We'll be at the airport to pick you and your bike up. This time you'll be feeling better, so we'll show you some of Charleston before you leave."

CHAPTER ELEVEN

South Atlantic Coast

The opulence of Florida's communities for wealthy retirees and executives is matched by the squalor and poverty of the migrant worker camps. It came home to us most clearly when one morning we toured the Kennedy Space Center facilities, where billions were being poured into the moon shots, and that same afternoon we saw a farm laborer's sick child, flies swarming around its little body, lying on a bed at the Old Top Labor Camp at Winter Haven.

—Neal R. Pierce and Jerry Hagstrom,
The Book of America

As I biked down the South Atlantic Coast, I noticed disturbing contrasts similar to those seen by Pierce and Hagstrom in Florida. At one moment I would be experiencing a Currier and Ives print of pastoral beauty and southern elegance, then, within a few miles, the scene might change to snarling dogs, rubbish-strewn roadside, and evidence of abject poverty.

🚲 🚲 🚲

On November 5, 1985, I left Charleston and headed south on U.S. 17 to resume my journey around the United States. A sign on the Edisto River bridge proclaimed "Welcome to South Carolina Low Country." Trucks loaded with thirty-two-foot pine logs roared past.

I rented a room at Edisto Motel, then rode back to the Edisto Nature Trail to identify shrubs and trees by reading the common and scientific names listed on signs along the trail. I was happy to make their acquaintance and enjoyed such southern-flavored names as persimmon, red buckeye, and pignut hickory.

After pedaling nine miles the next morning, I microwaved a sausage and bun and enjoyed a cup of coffee at the Woodstock Campground and Store. The rhythm of the road was returning. A brisk headwind, the morning cold, and the challenge of staying alive on a rough, heavily traveled highway sharpened my senses. Logging trucks came disturbingly close to my body. There was little room for the trucks to move over and I couldn't expect them to stop or slow while I found a place to pull out. It was a risk of the road I willingly took.

I couldn't resist stopping to read historic site signs. At one I read:

On top of this ridge stood a sylvan temple erected before the Revolution by Colonel Barnard Elliott, patriot and sportsman. The structure was supported by columns in the classic manner. The site, a part of Col. Elliott's plantation, Bellview, afforded an excellent stand for hunting deer.

Recalling chilly hours in primitive duck blinds and on crudely constructed stands while hunting white-tailed deer, I was amazed at such deluxe accommodations for hunting.

Five miles down the highway, I noticed twelve vultures circling overhead. Two miles later, joined by five more fellow scavengers, they were following, still circling. I hoped they didn't know something I didn't!

Ann Close, the Alfred A. Knopf editor who helped so much with my book *Above Timberline,* had suggested I visit her mother, Bea Lane, in Bluffton. When I arrived, Bea and her husband, Pres, offered to take me to Hilton Head, a barrier island that "formed" rather than split off from the mainland as do most of the coastal islands. Formed islands, Pres told me, are more likely to have fauna and flora not found on the mainland. He described them as *"really a new creation."* I liked that. But I didn't like other creations that were new. They reminded me of rapidly developing "stacked condominiums" in the Aspen and Vail areas of Colorado. Bea called the Florida condominiums "stack shacks."

We passed several fast food places. Nearby, a security guard warned that it was impossible to get to the beach in this area because of private communities.

Lagoons encircled some luxury homes. Bea told me alligators in some lagoons provided extra protection.

This area along South Carolina's coast was settled by the Scots in pre-Revolution days. A delightful and knowledgeable descendant, Temple McTeer, guided our private tour of the Waddell Mariculture Research and Development Center. A major activity here was to develop farming techniques for marine and brackish-water species of fish, mollusks, crustaceans, and plants.

After crossing the Savannah River into Georgia, I inquired at Jiffy's convenience store about any restaurants ahead. "I've heard about the Ritz in Garden City. Is that a restaurant?" I asked.

"Well, yes, but I don't think you'll want to go there," an attractive woman offered.

Puzzled, I asked, "Don't they serve food?"

"Yes," she responded, "but it's sort of a pub."

"That's okay. I'll want a beer anyway."

"Well, okay, but that's where all the blacks hang out."

So that was it! "Isn't it all right for me to go, even if the others there are black?" I asked.

"Sure, but I thought you might be a little uncomfortable."

I thanked her for her thoughtfulness and wondered how I would feel as a lone black in an all-white community.

I inquired about a motel and a man suggested Carole's. After riding a couple of miles to the motel, I had paid for the room when this same black man drove up. "Just wanted to see if you made it okay and got a room."

In the first two hours on the road next morning, twenty logging trucks passed me. Many were more considerate of my right to share the road than the logging truck drivers in Michigan, Maine, and the Pacific Northwest. They slowed, pulled over, usually smiled, and gave a wave or friendly beep. I felt guilty when one truck driver slowed to my pace up a long hill and waited for a wide enough place to pass without forcing me off the no-shoulder road.

A man with blaze orange jacket and camouflage fatigues was standing by a pickup. I asked if he was hunting deer. "Yes," he answered, "The three-month season began on October twentieth."

Later, along a ninety-mile stretch of State Highway 121, many pickups in turnouts or side roads were surrounded by men dressed in blaze orange jackets and camouflage trousers. I stopped to talk with four of these hunting parties. Each party had one or two cages of Walker hounds and was well supplied with a cooler of beer and one or more bottles of booze.

They were hunting white-tailed deer and told me that most hunters in this area belonged to hunting clubs that leased hunting privileges from timber companies. Radios were used to help locate the deer and get hunters and dogs to them. After a kill, they called someone to bring a vehicle as close as possible to reduce carrying or dragging the deer out of the woods. Radios were useful too, they claimed, to keep track of the dogs and keep hunters from getting lost.

One group of hunters included a father and his ten-year-old son. The father explained that the boy had gotten straight A's and as a reward, his dad had taken him out of school to "learn how to hunt and be a man." All I saw or heard was talking on the radio, drinking beer, and swapping stories spiced with profanity, obscenities, and sexually explicit comments. The boy's embarrassment was apparent. I sensed his relief when one of the hounds took off down the highway and a hunter yelled, "Hey, kid, go fetch that sonofabitch."

I didn't perceive much manliness or tutoring of the boy to become a good hunter in any of this. Of course, I readily admit that, in addition to incidents observed during this bicycle trek, many experiences during my years as a hunter and as a field biologist working with hunters have led to cynicism about some of the values touted for hunting as it is often done today.

Make no mistake. I recognize that hunting is often an important tool to maintain healthy wildlife populations in healthy habitats. But hunters, as a group, need to improve their conduct and ethics, and reassess their techniques.

🚲 🚲 🚲

At White Oak, I turned southeast on State Highway 252 and was in back-woods Georgia. Almost immediately, three dogs were snarling at wheels, pedals, and my legs. One sounded like he had missed breakfast.

A few mobile homes were scattered back in the pine timber. Most homes were unpainted shacks with trademark rusty tin roofs. Huge piles of garbage and trash surrounded houses.

Of six cars in front of a small shack, only three appeared operational. The yard was further decorated with a junked refrigerator, a battered stove, and assorted pots and pans—a scene typical for miles. More than half the vehicles rumbling down the highway were pickups. Most of the cars were Mercurys, Pontiacs, or other large sedans of 1960s or early 1970s vintage.

Two black ladies stood near a shack where a stovepipe protruded from a wall and smoke ascended lazily in the humid air. Stopping, I asked, "Why does the stovepipe come out of the wall instead of the roof?"

After scrutinizing me for several seconds, one responded with an answer so logical I felt embarrassed for having asked: "'Cause it's the shortest way out."

In early afternoon I picked up my mail in Folkston. Deciding to read and respond to the mail in a comfortable setting, I got a room in the Georgian Motel two miles out of town. A recently widowed man and his five sons, aged seventeen to twenty-eight, had taken over the motel five weeks earlier. Their enthusiasm for improving the buildings and updating services was evident.

The next day I pitched my tent on dry needles under a pine tree in a KOA campground near the entrance to Okefenokee National Wildlife Refuge. The Okefenokee Swamp is actually a vast peat bog so unstable in places that it trembles when stepped upon. The name is derived from the Choctaw Indian word meaning "quivering earth."

I unloaded the bike and pitched my gear inside the tent, then biked to the Suwannee Canal Recreation Area. There, I joined a boat tour, and, as we glided through the Suwannee Canal dug in 1891, the tour guide told us that during a drought in 1954 the swamp forest burned for eleven months, resulting in what he called "prairies." These now appeared as vast expanses of dark but highly reflective water, lush with colorful blooms and dotted with "hammocks" on which shrubs and trees have taken root.

Along the canal banks were bald cypress trees, with their grotesquely picturesque "knees." Also lining the banks were gum and huge-leaved red bay trees with streamers of Spanish moss. An understory of red-berried Cassena holly and yellow-flowered Titi bushes provided a riotous diversity of color and form. I photographed a large alligator, one of the 10,000 to 12,000 the guide said reside in the Okefenokee Swamp.

After the boat tour, I biked to the Chesser Island Homestead and found Vannie Chesser rocking on the spacious front porch. She counted me as the day's seventy-third visitor with a click of her "tally whacker."

Next morning, I crossed the Saint Mary's River, which drains the Okefenokee into the Atlantic and marks the boundary between Georgia and Florida. At Macclenny, I turned east into a steady headwind on U.S. 90, a rough two-lane road. The ditches on both sides were filled with stagnant water, beer cans and bottles, plastic containers, cardboard boxes, discarded utensils, and equipment.

The scenery changed quickly, however, in the first block of Baldwin City. Five large handsome homes, surrounded by manicured one- to two-acre grounds were guarded by high chain-link fences and snarling dogs that charged the fence as if they wanted a piece of me. Another example of a "fortress mentality" held by some affluent Americans? A large American flag hung limply in the damp air from a pole in each front yard.

Suddenly I was in a sleazy business district. Lloyd's Package Liquor Store. Whiskey and cold beer advertised in windows on opposite corners of an intersection. Pool hall. "Movieland Video, Over 2,800 Titles." Fast food places. A BLT sandwich was all I figured I could trust at Everybody's Cafe. While it was being prepared, I visited the filthiest restroom encountered south of Charleston and returned to the greasiest BLT I ever tried to eat.

For the last fifteen miles to Jacksonville, I pushed the pedals hard into increasing headwinds. First task at the Sunshine Inn was to spread out damp tent, sleeping bag, and other gear.

☙ ☙ ☙

A sheriff parked alongside U.S. 17 south of Orange Park, motioned for me to stop. First, he chatted about hair-raising experiences with motorists when riding his motorcycle in this country. Then he asked, "Aren't you worried about people on the road? That's the only thing that would bother me. With all the crazies around this country, I wouldn't want to be alone on a bicycle." I heard many comments like this. I just couldn't worry about them.

☙ ☙ ☙

A local couple, about my age, were sitting on old chairs in the corner of a roadside country store. They asked about my trip. The man remarked, "My wife and I often talk about doing something like you're doing. We sure envy you."

I empathized with their yearnings, assured them that such an adventure was within their capabilities, and urged them to follow their dreams.

Sweating down U.S. 17, I thought about the couple back in the store. They looked a lot more comfortable and less tired than I felt, though I'm not sure that they were. At times when not getting much serious exercise, I have often felt lethargic or downright tired. When I am on the road riding hard all day, I have more energy and enthusiasm. After getting into a motel or camp-ground, taking a hot shower, having a cold beer or glass of wine and a good dinner, I feel terrific. And life seems great, even after hurting a good share of the day.

I saw road kills in various stages of decomposition. First an armadillo, then two hounds, then an opossum, then two more armadillos and another hound. A raccoon ended my body count a few miles north of Saint Augustine.

Despite the scavenger banquets viewed along the highway, I arrived at Scottish Inn in Saint Augustine with a hearty appetite. The loquacious and well-informed waitress let me know "right off" that Saint Augustine was our nation's oldest city. It was founded in 1565 by Spanish Admiral Don Pedro Menendez de Aviles. For centuries the city served as the capital of colonial Florida. A more recent fact, she told me, was that Robert L. Ripley, known "hereabouts" as the modern Marco Polo, traveled to 198 countries to gather 750 exhibits. These were now displayed in Saint Augustine's "very own" Believe-It-Or-Not Museum.

Next morning, I saw the ocean for the first time since leaving Charleston. Awesome! Huge waves rolled in nearly to the highway. Fog soft-ly blanketed the landscape with an ethereal beauty. A man and woman float-ed slowly past in the fog. Walking on the beach, I supposed, but only their upper bodies were visible.

At 7:15 A.M. I pulled off the highway to wipe rearview mirror, map case, odometer, and glasses. It wasn't hot or raining, but the humidity was 100 per-cent and my biking clothes and bare legs were sopping wet. Cars had lights on and windshield wipers swished off the moisture.

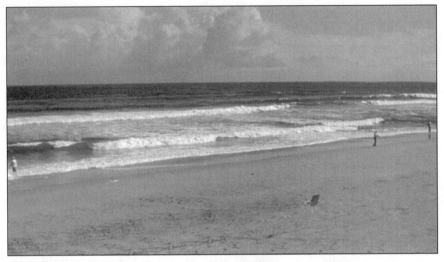

I saw the ocean for the first time since leaving Charleston. Awesome!

At the Dolphin Restaurant south of Saint. Augustine, Chris Burden, a director of Marineland, said he had passed me while driving to work that morning and invited me to join him for breakfast. His father was the first president of Marineland when it opened in 1938, he said. As Chris stopped to pay, the cashier looked at me and exclaimed, "Hey, I saw you on your bicycle about three miles north of here as I came to work."

Chris then escorted me to the Marineland administration building where he introduced me to the current president, Dave Drysdale. Dave called Bill Pucket, director of marketing and public relations, and asked him to take me on a walking tour of Marineland "for as long as it takes."

It took about two hours, was a good break from long days of biking, and gave me a chance to take some interesting photos. My favorite was one at the dolphin tank where a man, suspended in a bucket over the tank, held a fish in each hand and one in his teeth. In choreographic synchronism, three dolphins leaped simultaneously to a height of sixteen feet and snatched the fish.

🚴   🚴   🚴

I shouted, "Whoopee!" squeezed the brakes and skidded to a stop as my odometer registered 10,000 miles. The summer before when I had completed the second leg of this journey, a newspaper reporter interviewed me. His article was headlined "Senior Pedals 10,000 Miles," though the actual mileage was only 9,549. Now I had earned that headline.

There were times of uncertainty, though, such as when logging trucks crowded me on narrow highways and I had no place to go, or when a drunk in an old pickup just missed me while his acid rock stereo blasted my eardrums. Each time I had thought, "another few inches and I would have been history." But 10,000 miles had a solid sound to it, and I had no doubt about finishing the ride.

After crossing Saint John's River, I saw a sign, "Central Florida State Zoological Park," and an abandoned entrance shelter beside an attractive side road. It looked appealing, so I took a detour that led to still another detour.

Paul and Jean Robinson, docents at the park, told me some of their adventures with a twenty-eight-foot sailboat Paul bought after retiring from thirty years with the navy.

After I mentioned wanting to fly along the Florida coast, Paul offered, "Jean and I have to lead a thirty-minute tour with a group of school kids. Look around the park, then we'll load your bike in our pickup and drive you to Sanford Airport." I called the airport to arrange to rent a Cessna 172.

Cutting through the smooth air was a pleasant diversion from pounding my butt on rough roads. Absorbed in flying and photographing the NASA Causeway across the Intracoastal Waterway, I quickly returned to reality when an authoritative voice barked into my headset, "Small aircraft approaching Cape Canaveral from the west. You are entering a restricted area. Execute a 180-degree turn immediately." Chastened, I realized I'd misread the flight chart. Obviously I needed more navigating experience. But I did get a recognizable photo of the Canaveral launch tower before turning!

In 550 miles traveled through South Carolina, Georgia, and northern Florida since leaving Charleston, nothing had interested me as a place to live until I was south of Orlando. Here, along County Road 15 between Narcoossee and Saint Cloud and east of East Lake Tohopekaliga were lovely homes in the community of Live Oaks. At a Burger King, I met a couple about my age who highly recommended Live Oaks as a place to live. Its cleanliness and beauty were impressive.

At Canoe Creek Campground my enthusiasm ebbed. I paid $11.24 to pitch my tent on a tiny patch of grass. Restroom and showers were dirty; the

picnic table had rotted. As I prepared to get in my sleeping bag, two men saun-
tered over. One asked, "Aren't you worried about snakes and spiders crawling
into your tent with you?"

"You aren't? Guess I'm just chicken, but I could never do that."

The other asked, "Carry a gun don't you?"

"You don't? Well, I sure wouldn't be without one on these roads where
all the rednecks carry rifles in their pickups and all these crazies are riding
motorcycles."

Then they chimed in together, "Well, we hope you have a good night."

That night I left the rain tarp off and the tent flaps open because, in the
past, high humidity had caused the tarp and tent to become soaked inside and
out. Despite these precautions, the tent was soaked outside and hundreds of
droplets of moisture glistened on the inside next morning. After turning the
tent inside out and shaking it violently, I finally rolled up the whole soggy mess
and strapped it across the back panniers.

As I pedaled down State Highway 523, subdued rays of sunlight emerged
above the eastern horizon to backlight cattle, horses, and white wooden
fences, standing ghostlike in the fog. Spanish moss streamed from the branches
of live oaks along the road. From time to time a great blue heron, snowy egret,
or an American bittern would rise silently, gracefully, from a water-filled
ditch. Hairs on my arms and legs were covered with silvery beads of water that
glowed in the misty half-light. A mystical morning. Breathing deeply, riding
smoothly, my feeling of being part of nature was enhanced by the deep,
musical murmur of sandhill cranes communicating as they wedged through
the overhanging fog.

When the sun finally broke through, I had biked fifteen miles and was
hungry. Calling from Fort Drum, I found that morning mass was at 10:30
A.M. at Sacred Heart Catholic Church in Okeechobee twelve miles ahead.
Plenty of time for a honey bun and coffee at the general store.

Carl, foreman of a nearby cattle ranch, sat beside me at the store counter.
He was just the person to answer my questions about the "strange" cattle I'd
seen. Carl told me those with big, floppy ears and long, wide-angled horns
were "Brangus," a Brahma/Black Angus cross. There was also a Brahma/
Hereford cross called "Braford." He explained that short, slick hair and other
physiological characteristics of the Brahma were better adapted to this hot,

humid country than were Black Angus and Herefords. But the latter breeds gave the cross better quality beef.

In Yeehaw Junction I listened to reports of hurricane-force winds approaching the mainland so I decided to push hard for Fort Meyers and hole up as long as necessary. Despite photo ops I couldn't pass by, attending mass in Okeechobee, visits with interesting people such as Carl, and increasing headwinds, I pedaled seventy-five miles to Moorehaven well before nightfall.

During breakfast Monday morning, I listened to forecasters debate whether Hurricane Kate would hit the Florida coast, then I hit the road. Rain and hard gusting winds were challenges as I biked sixty miles to Palm City Motel in Fort Meyers. Amazed I was riding in this weather, the manager cleaned out a storage room for my bike and helped put all my gear in a room.

Old Faithful and I were ready to see what would happen in our first encounter with a hurricane.

CHAPTER TWELVE

Gulf of Mexico

A Mercury sedan has advantages over a Specialized Expedition bicycle when traveling at the edge of a hurricane. Soft music on the radio soothes as fierce winds contort the trees wildly and I sit in air-conditioned comfort while keeping a firm grip on the steering wheel.

—from my taped journal

The weather forecast promised rainsqualls and heavy winds for a couple of days. I had rented an auto and would use Palm City Motel as base camp for exploring the southern tip of Florida.

South of Fort Meyers I found a photographer's paradise while walking a boardwalk that provided access to the Fakahatchee Strand in Big Cypress Swamp, a flat, gently sloping limestone plain. During the rainy season, water flows slowly southward into the mangrove swamps bordering the Gulf of Mexico. Over time the water has cut channels in the limestone. These are now bordered by tall, dense swamp forests called "strands." The Fakahatchee is twenty miles long and three to five miles wide.

Although logging, drainage, and fires have negatively impacted natural values, threatened or endangered remnant populations of the wood stork, Florida black bear, mangrove fox squirrel, Everglades mink, and the Florida panther remain.

It was hard to believe that all these creatures were tenacious enough to survive in this dank environment of bald cypress, royal palms, strangler figs, and algae-covered swamp water. But I could appreciate the wild mystery of the place and realized that I knew little about these habitats.

A three-mile causeway led to the Ding Darling National Wildlife Refuge on Sanibel Island. The refuge was named after Jay Norwood Darling, who signed "Ding" on his political cartoons which won Pulitzer Prizes in 1923 and 1942. Darling, who headed the U.S. Biological Survey (now the Fish and Wildlife Service) during Franklin Roosevelt's administration, was a key person in establishing the national wildlife refuge system. Another of his contributions to wildlife was the initiation, in 1934, of the Migratory Bird Hunting Stamp program, for which he designed the first stamp. Proceeds from these stamps have purchased 186 national wildlife refuges.

Wildlife species along a five-mile drive in the refuge provided a festival of colors: the bright pink roseate spoonbill, brown pelican, white ibis, black double-crested cormorant with its metallic green head, and yellow-crowned night heron with large orange eyes. The anhinga, glossy black with silver wing patches, should have been a circus performer. It dives underwater where it spears a fish with its long, slender bill, then comes to the surface and tosses the fish into midair and swallows it head first.

After leaving the refuge, I drove around this twelve-mile-long subtropical barrier island with its mangrove swamps and white sandy beaches. Though the main force of Hurricane Kate had passed, high winds made driving unpleasant so I parked in a somewhat protected cove, opened a refuge brochure, and sat in the car reading about the Calusa Indians who used the island as a place to live and find food more than 2,000 years ago. Farming and fishing provided a living for European settlers from the mid-1800s until 1926 when a hurricane destroyed their agricultural pursuits. Tourism is now the economic foundation for island residents.

My stomach told me that it was time to come back to the present, so I drove to McT's Shrimp House and Tavern. The evening special was broiled blacktail shark with an excellent sauce and a catchy description: "Shiver me timbers. It's a change of plot. You eat the shark."

Back in the saddle again after a two-day concession to Hurricane Kate, I left Palm City Motel early and quickly discovered that riding a bicycle requires more skill and guts than tooling a Mercury down the same highway. It had rained the previous night so the pavement was wet and treacherous. Riding over the Caloosahatchie River on a narrow sidewalk elevated above the traffic, I saw an accumulation of glass—too late. Then I pushed the bike a mile to Tireland at 300 Pondella Road, where owner Frank Shore would replace the rear tire and tube.

On the way I had stopped to ask directions from two friendly barbers with no customers. They wanted to talk. After asking about the bike trip, one commented, "With all the rough characters across the country, it seems you would be in constant fear that something drastic would happen to you." That concern again!

Convinced these warnings of dire consequences were mostly projections of people's own fears, I shrugged off negative thoughts, mounted Old Faithful, and headed northwest along the gulf.

A snowy egret decided to join me for a while. This striking bird was ahead, standing in tall grass about twenty-five feet off the highway. When I approached, it sprang into the air and flew a hundred yards before landing again. This went on for more than a mile before the egret finally perched in a pine tree and let me pass.

While taking a Gatorade break at a convenience store a couple of miles south of Punta Gorda, I met Dr. Richard Wingert and his wife, Kay. Richard is an ear,

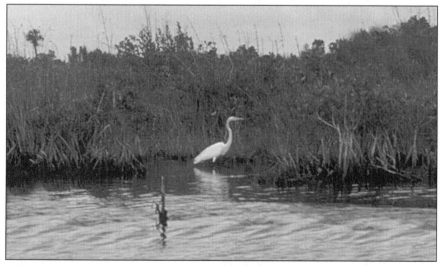

As I bicycled closer, this snowy egret sprang into the air and flew about a hundred yards before landing again. This went on for more than a mile until, finally, it perched in a pine tree and let me pass.

nose, and throat specialist. Both are competitive runners and engage in other out-door activities. While Richard was doing his residency in Tacoma, Washington, they hiked and climbed mountains in the northern Cascades. The Pacific Northwest enchanted them, but they didn't much care for southern Florida. Richard called it the obesity capital of the world. He said, "Many people here are old, wealthy, and self-indulgent. Doctors too often pander to their weaknesses."

When Richard and Kay had run earlier this morning, the temperature was eighty degrees, the humidity 99 percent. Richard commented, "Under those conditions, you don't have much get-up-and-go." But they got up and went, as their enthusiasm and firmly chiseled bodies attested.

As I straddled my bike, ready to stand on the pedals and start moving the heavy load, Richard squeezed my hand and blurted, "Just a minute. I've got a great idea. We live on a quiet island. You can stay a couple of days with us and rest up. We'll show you around this part of Florida." The offer was tempting, but I moved on.

Seven miles north of Venice, I stopped for breakfast at the Travis Family Restaurant and met Bob Ladley. Bob was my age, had bicycled several "centuries" (100 miles in a day), and had just begun flying lessons. He told of a local newspaper story warning cyclists about "grabbers," usually young guys in a pickup who slow, pull in close, then hit or grab at the rider. Others throw things at you, Bob said. Once he received a severe bruise on his left calf from a thrown beer bottle. Lots of folks called him an old fool because he rode U.S. 41 where numerous bicycle accidents had occurred.

ۼ ۼ ۼ

At Big Oak Trailer Park and Campground three miles north of Masaryktown, I pitched my tent in the grassy space next to Joe Legendre's trailer. Eighty-three years old, Joe had twenty-one grandchildren and twenty-eight great-grandchildren. He had been a mailman for thirty-seven years. For most of those years, Joe walked an eighteen- to twenty-two-mile route. It must have been good for him. He was wiry, quick moving, sharp as a tack, and until he told me his age, I judged him to be about sixty-five. A lifelong Catholic, Joe had lost his wife eleven years prior and attributed his good health, good humor, and positive outlook on life to his faith and the support of friends. He lived in Derry, New Hampshire, about six months of the year and spent winters at Big Oak Trailer Park.

The next morning Joe's door opened while I lashed tent, sleeping bag, and foam pad atop my panniers. The tantalizing aroma of fresh-brewed coffee and frying bacon caused me to turn as Joe called out, "Come in for a cup of coffee while I start the pancakes and eggs."

Joe had seen me breaking camp and quickly started breakfast so I could join him. As I reflect back on this journey, it is clear that many of my treasured memories came from such spontaneous friendliness and generosity.

In Archer I stayed overnight with Tim and June O'Meara, former students at Colorado State University who were expecting me. The next morning, Tim, a biological scientist at the University of Florida in Gainesville, drove me to Gainesville for breakfast with Wayne Marion, also a former CSU student and now an associate professor of wildlife ecology. Later, I rented a Cessna 172 at Gainesville Airport; then Wayne described local landscapes as we headed south over Payne's Prairie, an 18,000-acre freshwater marsh.

We flew along the western boundary of Ocala National Forest, known for great stands of sand pine, many winding streams, and more than 600 lakes. Wayne told me that the Ocala is home to Florida's state bird, the northern mockingbird. Having Wayne point out the diverse ecosystems and explain their interrelationships added to my enjoyment and knowledge as we cruised at 130 miles per hour over the landscape.

♲ ♲ ♲

Between Mayo and the Fenholloway River, a Toyota pickup carrying two hunters in the cab and two boys and two hounds in the back, slowed beside me. One hunter called, "We sure hope you have a nice trip and wish you well." As they speeded up, all four gave a big wave and the hounds wagged their tails. Better for morale than an early morning caffeine fix.

For the first hour after leaving Gandy Motor Lodge in Perry the next morning, I pedaled in fog so heavy I couldn't see seventy-five feet. The blinking beacon protected my behind. I hoped.

One to two feet of water languished under trees and shrubs on both sides of the highway, the result of recent heavy rains. Fifty feet off the highway, a hunters' camp boasted four tents, all surrounded by water. Obscured in this swampy, foggy environment, I could hear hounds baying and guns barking. I hoped the hunters could see their targets.

The 130 miles on U.S. 98 from Perry to Newport, then northwest on State Highway 267 through the Apalachicola National Forest to Bloxham, I remember mostly for fog, intermittent heavy rainstorms, and pine trees.

Around Blountstown hundreds of pines had been snapped off ten to twenty feet above the ground during Hurricane Kate. It reminded me of pine forests in Germany devastated by artillery shells, both theirs and ours, in World War II.

A 1.7-mile-long bridge over the Apalachicola River broke my reverie. No shoulder. Heavy traffic. I didn't recognize the problem until well onto the bridge when a trucker pulled up behind me. A steady stream of oncoming traffic kept him from passing. I had no place to go except ahead. Spin the pedals! Even so, the line of cars behind me became impressively long. No one signaled their impatience, though they had good cause. Once off the bridge I pulled onto the shoulder and saluted my appreciation as they passed.

Pedaling on a wet highway while dodging armadillo roadkills hadn't been a lot of fun. But, no doubt about it, grinding out seventy-eight miles of adrenaline-inducing miles was better than any sleeping pill for assuring a good night's sleep at the Cannon Motel in Panama City that night.

Next morning I set my watch one hour back and moved into the Central Time Zone. The temperature had dropped to forty degrees and a cold wind was blowing out of the north. After only three miles, hot coffee and an omelet breakfast was welcome. A man at the next table nodded toward Old Faithful and asked, "Is that your Cadillac parked out front?" Ran Humphries and his wife, Ann, owned the Ageless Bookstore in Panama City and Ran was president of Allied Business Machines.

We visited for a half hour. Ran remarked that two types of people were migrating into the gulf area of Florida. Wealthy retirees were creating a market for big luxury condos and other businesses. "Of course, that is good for the local economy, but the sand dunes are being destroyed in the process," Ran added.

"Another type of people came to Florida to avoid paying property, income, and sales taxes," he said. They were retired but not wealthy. They contributed little to the economy because their purpose was to enjoy the winter climate while spending little.

"They live in trailer villages, mobile home courts, campgrounds, or low-cost motels. You have to respect their desire to have a place in the sun," Ran remarked, "but they are not a positive economic force in Florida."

As they left, Ran picked up my bill and brushed aside my protests with, "Wish we could do more for someone undertaking an adventure like yours."

On the road again in heavy traffic, I failed to realize I was approaching another high, narrow bridge. There was no place to get out of the traffic. It had happened again. I had to dig in and hope for the best. For 0.7 miles cars had to slow behind me. A few zipped around when there was a gap in traffic. No one beeped or showed impatience. Still, I breathed a sigh of relief when I exited the bridge and was on a narrow shoulder again.

A mile later I needed to turn left onto the scenic route along the beaches. I was on the shoulder with two lanes of fast, tailgating traffic between me and the left turn exit. Checking the rearview mirror, I spotted a tiny "hole" in the nearest lane, signaled, rolled into the space, checked the mirror again. No hole in the next lane to the left! Remembering my friend Hartley's advice to ride assertively, I vigorously jabbed my left arm outward until an overtaking car in that lane began slowing. Without hesitation, I maxed quad power and shot in ahead of him, signaled again, then turned left onto Alternate Route 98. Whew!

A few miles later a car passed slowly and stopped on the shoulder. The driver got out and motioned for me to stop. It was Ran who had bought my breakfast. "My wife and I have been talking about you. We remembered you were taking this scenic route so decided to look for you and invite you to come back to our home. We have extra cars. You can take one to shop, sightsee, or do whatever you want. But we'd like to show you more of the country, take you out to dinner, and have you stay overnight. Tomorrow morning, we'll have an early breakfast and you can be on your way. What do you say?"

For a minute I couldn't say anything. Then I thought of my itinerary and the need to ride hard for Houston in order to meet commitments. Interpreting my hesitancy as being uncomfortable to stay in a stranger's home, Ran continued, "I have contacts with motels here in Panama City and along the gulf as you head west. I would be privileged to have you be my guest at any one of the motels."

The feelings that welled up in my heart were much larger than gratitude. My unexpected encounters with Ran and his wife stirred me. I had become more than a spectator. As a recipient of such openness and generosity, I had become a participant in the true spirit of America. It was hard to tell this kind man, average in stature but huge in spirit, that I had to hurry because I'd promised to fly north from Houston in time to spend Christmas with my son in Atlanta and New Year's Eve with Elisabeth in East Lansing.

🚲   🚲   🚲

Nineteen-year-old Hugh Evans of Berkeley, California, overtook me west of Panama City on Alternate Route 98. Hugh was traveling the United States wherever his imagination and bicycle took him. In three months this combination had taken him more than 3,200 miles. We chatted beside the highway for a half hour. Hugh had bought a Myata frame and high-quality components, then spent his spare time for two years customizing his bike. Besides fenders and four Cannondale low-rider panniers, his imagination held sway as he added an eclectic assortment of gadgets. On the front fender he mounted a miniature biplane with a propeller that spun as he rode. On the back hung a white Halloween mask and his bike-racing helmet. He preferred, he told me, to ride bareheaded so "I can feel the wind blowing in my hair." I suppressed the urge to lecture him on the importance of wearing, not carrying, a helmet.

With Plexiglas and heavy tape, he had fashioned two cones and attached one on each front pannier. He claimed they made a tremendous difference when going into a headwind. They must. He was only about five foot seven and couldn't weigh more than 125 pounds soaking wet. Yet he averaged seventy miles a day while "just taking it easy."

He admitted that he left Berkeley with negative stereotypes about people he would meet while crossing Texas. "But I was wrong," he grinned. "Almost all my experiences have been just great!" I could understand why.

After I had turned onto Alternate Route 98, much of the scenery consisted of billboards and signs. A few short stretches of gorgeous white sand beaches broke the ugly monotony.

"Navarre Baptist Church. Let us give thanks to the Lord" proclaimed a large sign. Nearby, a larger, higher, more garish sign read "Wards. Open 06:00.

Breakfast. Hamburgers, chili dogs, chili burgers, homemade root beer." A mile later, a huge Holiday Inn sign towered over the neighboring pines. The small, attractive, unobtrusive, informative business signs along New England highways were but a wistful memory.

After crossing Navarre Beach Bridge to Santa Rosa Island, I turned west and followed State Highway 399 along this barrier island. It seemed abandoned. Most of the homes, many built atop eight- to twelve-foot stilts, were unoccupied. Trash was strewn everywhere. Empty, battered garbage cans were under houses, on racks, or rolling in the wind. Sand blew across the road. Boardwalks stretched across sandy wasteland to empty beaches.

Suddenly, I realized I was humming "Waltzing Matilda," the theme song for *On the Beach,* a 1959 movie starring Gregory Peck, Fred Astaire, Anthony Perkins, and Ava Gardner. They were on a submarine and didn't know that a nuclear holocaust had wiped out the world's population until they surfaced near Australia and found a deserted land. Santa Rosa Island reminded me of that movie's lonely, eerie setting.

🚲 🚲 🚲

The sign on the Perdido River bridge read "Welcome to Alabama the Beautiful."

Three hunters with "Lillian Swamp Hunting Club" embossed across the front of their blaze orange caps told me that the hunting season was open for white-tailed deer, raccoon, cottontails, doves, and northern bobwhites.

I turned onto Baldwin County Highway 62 West and for several miles. Hereford and Black Angus beef cattle grazed in lush pastures surrounded by fences built with white-painted wooden planks. Farmers were cultivating rich-looking soil in neatly fenced fields. Attractive brick or brick-and-frame homes were surrounded by large yards, often with manicured shrubs in front and nice lawns dotted with pine trees around sides and back. After enjoying these bucolic scenes, I was surprised when locals told me how tough farming was in the area. They said the only ones making any money were those growing "wacky weed."

A few miles later a small country store presented another contrast. The large glass windows in front were protected by five-eighths-inch reinforced steel bars about four inches apart. Outside the regular door, two outer doors were constructed with heavy steel bars. A heavy chain and padlock hung from one, ready to lock them together.

I asked the couple inside, "Does this place function part time as the jail?"

Without taking offense, the man replied, "Well, with the kind of people around here, you learn to protect yourself. Where you goin' on that bike?"

"To Mobile," I responded.

They both shook their heads. "It'll be dark before you get there," the man said. "And it's a bad enough neighborhood to go through in broad daylight. Boats drop drugs off all along the coast. Anything you've heard about drugs is worse here. We don't want to worry you, but we would never feel right if we didn't warn you."

I thanked them for the warning and told them I'd stayed out of trouble so far.

An hour later a couple of young fellows in a van slowed beside me while one yelled, "Get yore ass off that bike, old man." I didn't know if they were going to stop and invite me to go a round or two, or if they just felt I needed a rest. In any event, I picked up the cadence a notch while warily watching for the van to return.

Fifteen minutes later most car headlights were on and I was in front of the Malbis Motel in Daphne. Deciding that discretion was the better part of valor, I checked in for the night.

The motel manager eagerly told of a local attraction, the magnificent classical Greek Orthodox Church. In a booklet, "The Faith of Jason Malbis," I read that a young monk named Antonios Markopoulos had migrated from Greece to America. Soon afterward, he legally changed his name to Jason Malbis. He was unskilled, unlettered, and destitute. He also was imbued with the teachings of the gospel and a dream to establish a Greek settlement and farming community.

Mr. Malbis's vision of a great church was not realized in his lifetime. He died in 1942; the Greek Orthodox Church was completed in 1965.

Next morning, I stopped at the church and a retired engineer who took care of the chimes, electrical systems, and anything mechanical that goes wrong unlocked the front door and turned on the lights. The Malbis church was copied after a church in Athens with the exacting details of Byzantine architecture and marble from the same quarry that provided stone for the Parthenon. More than 150 paintings of religious figures and biblical scenes graced the walls and seventy-five-foot domed ceiling, my self-appointed guide told me as I photographed some of them.

Twelve miles later I crossed the Admiral Raphael Semmes Bridge and was in Benville Square, a park surrounded by businesses in the center of Old Mobile. Hollis Johnston, a custodian in the square, told me that the park was established in 1824. He warned me that people in Benville Square couldn't be trusted. I am glad this old black man was honest, because he watched Old Faithful for a couple of hours while I took photos and talked with people loafing in the square.

A few miles south of Mobile, I had a number of close calls in heavy traffic. A pickup swerved near me and the driver yelled, "Get that damn bicycle off the street!"

In a following van, a scruffy-looking girl screamed, "Take your fuckin' bike off this road!" as she barely missed my left elbow.

It was worth all the trouble, however, when I arrived at Bellingrath Gardens. Walter and Bessie Morse Bellingrath had acquired the property in 1918 for a private fishing lodge. But the primeval setting inspired them to develop one of the most renowned gardens in the world. It was opened to the public in 1932.

At the entrance building, a charming black woman moved nursery carts so I could lean my bicycle inside where it would be safe. She listened to the story of my ride, then paid my four-dollar admittance ticket, saying I was her guest and asking me to send her a card when I got home.

The tranquil beauty of landscaping, the presence of myriad species of singing birds, and the charm of design and construction of buildings created an almost spiritual atmosphere. I later read in a brochure that Bellingrath's belief in the importance of "the spiritual life as a fundamental part of the educational process" led him to establish a foundation that provides financial support for three colleges and two churches.

🚲 🚲 🚲

I rode into Mississippi on U.S. 90 late in the afternoon. For more than a century, this stretch of coast was a summer playground for Old South gentility and a winter vacation spot for Midwesterners. Gulf-front mansions and luxurious resort hotels were built and surrounded by moss-covered oaks and magnolia trees. This all changed with World War II. A shipbuilding industry and oil refineries at Pascagoula ushered in a new industrial flavor. This region of Mississippi's Gulf Coast is now described in *The Book of America* as "a fast-growing 'strip city' between Mobile and New Orleans."

Framed by my camera lens in addition to the sign "Pascagoula Corp Limits" was a column of unsightly power lines marching down a weedy, littered median. Telephone lines, shoddy buildings, and gaudy billboards visually debased the sides of the highway. In the same photo the setting sun blushed in radiant glory beneath a huge billboard that towered above adjacent trees.

From Pascagoula I had followed U.S. 90 west for forty-six miles when a light sprinkle caused me to shield the lens while photographing stately antebellum homes in Pass Christian; then it turned into a downpour. I pedaled quickly to the Rusty Pelican Restaurant and ordered my first-ever Creole gumbo. Hot! Spicy! Delicious! I savored the gumbo, then ordered a dish of ice cream and a cup of coffee to delay becoming soaking wet again. Glad I did because Mr. Royce Hill, vice president and general manager of Heritage Investment Corporation, came in and ordered a cup of coffee. "Mind if I pull up a chair and join you?" he asked.

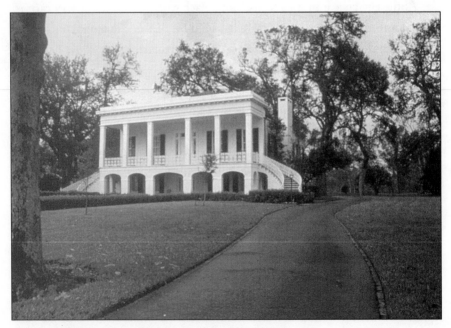

A stately antebellum home in Pass Christian, Mississippi

We discussed options for continuing down the coast. Royce advised me to turn onto Pass Christian's Scenic Drive, which climbed to a low bluff overlooking the Gulf of Mexico. There I would see about fifty huge homes, most painted white and with wide verandas and tall colonnades, often on the second story. Enormous stately trees dominated the spacious lawns. These photogenic homes were fronted by fences, some white-painted wood, others elegant wrought iron.

Royce told me that in the 1920s and 1930s wealthy ladies and gentlemen had come into this area and purchased fashionable old homes for a few thousand dollars. Prices now ranged from $200,000 to well over $1 million. He could remember when there were gazebos along the beach where the gentility lounged on lawn chairs while sipping mint juleps. They would drive Model T Fords, and more expensive makes of that vintage, up and down the hard-packed beach as they stopped to visit or have a drink with their neighbors. Apparently, they were little affected by the Great Depression.

Royce obviously cherished memories of "the good old days." He claimed that Pass Christian retained more of the Old South than anywhere else between Mobile and New Orleans.

I stayed two nights in the Payless Motel near Waveland to avoid incessant downpours. One day was spent in the city library researching this region's fascinating history.

🚲 🚲 🚲

As I left Mississippi on U.S. 90, there were no houses for miles. Water edged the highway most of the time. In the distance I often heard hounds baying. Close up, frogs croaked loudly. Occasionally muddy side roads disappeared into the sodden forest. A quarter mile before crossing the Pearl River into Louisiana, I read "Unlawful to Track Mud on Highways." I wondered how could one get on the highway without tracking mud.

Despite wool gloves and heavy socks, my hands and feet were cold as I rode into Louisiana and, soon, into the corporate limits of New Orleans. In the next nine miles, I crossed three bridges, passed a goat tethered knee deep in muddy water, and counted three road-killed opossums.

During the last fifteen miles, rain continued, wind picked up, and the temperature dropped. Along the way I somehow wandered onto a horrendous access road and had to push through a strip of tall, wet grass to get back on the highway. Three miles before reaching the Quality Inn, I met the final challenge for the day on a long, narrow bridge that forced heavy traffic into a single lane.

What to do? I grabbed the handlebars tight, gritted my teeth, tightened my sphincter, and assertively signaled a left turn while glancing in the rearview mirror. When the driver immediately behind me hesitated, I shot into the tiny space and endured incessant beeping by impatient drivers until I had cleared the end of the bridge. Wet, cold, and miserable, I crossed that damn bridge without a flicker of fear. But, as the danger diminished, the familiar euphoric feeling told me adrenaline had been pumping like mad.

Two hours later I was in the Marina Wharf Restaurant sipping a glass of Blue Nun, a favorite wine in these parts, and enjoying Chef Bienvenue, fried oysters on English muffins smothered with hollandaise sauce.

The next morning, I turned west on the Saint Bernard Highway and reached the city limits of New Orleans, after riding 28.5 miles inside the corporate limits. Riding along South Peter Street I saw a large white boat with three decks and a huge red paddlewheel on the stern anchored off the bank of the Mississippi River. I had stumbled, my usual technique for discovery, onto an authentic paddlewheeler, the *Creole Queen*.

The street was only yards away from the water, so I pedaled slowly, looking up at the boat towering beside Poydras Street Wharf. A man dressed in a natty blue uniform stood on the promenade deck. Using a megaphone he called down, "Where are you heading on that bicycle?"

Looking around and seeing no other bike, I shouted back, "San Diego!"

"Where have you ridden from?"

"Fort Collins, Colorado."

"Holy Mary, Mother of God! Well, push that bike up the gangplank and be my guest for a Mississippi River cruise."

When Old Faithful and I had reached the top of the gangplank, a cruise photographer took our picture and a young lady in crisp nautical attire said, "Hello there. I'm Reneé. Cap'n says for me to help you store your bike. Follow me."

The gangplank came up and the boat left the dock. I had just made the scheduled 10:00 A.M. departure.

We moved slowly as Reneé parted the tourists with "Excuse us, please." Our destination was one of the three Victorian-decorated dining rooms, the King's Room, where we leaned Old Faithful against the piano.

"Cap'n says you are to come up to the wheelhouse. He wants to visit with you."

A passageway led to the wheelhouse, but ended at a closed door with the sign "No Unauthorized Personnel Beyond This Point." Opening the door, I called, "May I come up?"

A friendly voice answered, "If you're the fellow on the bicycle, come on up."

There were two cocaptains on the cruise that day. We visited about my trip, about New Orleans and the Mississippi River, and they suggested ways to avoid dangerous neighborhoods on my way out of the city. As I left the wheelhouse, the one who had invited me extended his hand and smiled, "Be sure to enjoy our luncheon and visit the bar. You're my guest."

When I ordered a drink in the bar, the steward waved aside my five-dollar bill, saying, "It's paid for. You're the captain's guest." Luncheon tickets were being sold in the dining room. When I took out my billfold again, a different steward reminded me I was the captain's guest.

As we cruised up the muddy Mississippi past the French Quarter, historic Jackson Square, and the site of the famous Battle of New Orleans, I was surprised how much history occurred within sight of the river. At least the captain's narrative made it seem so. Especially enjoyable was our stop and walk to the old Beauregard House, a plantation mansion built seventeen years after Jackson's victory of 1815.

🚲 🚲 🚲

It took the next two days to bike to Franklin, 111 miles to the west. Not good time, but biking conditions were not good either. Mostly, I rode U.S. 90. Its oystershell shoulders were strewn with debris and difficult to ride. Often, vehicles were hauling sugarcane and left an obstacle course of stalks and mud, made even slicker by intermittent rain. A steady stream of impatient, speeding, horn-honking motorists added to the dangerous conditions.

The Forest Restaurant in Franklin, Louisiana, offered a tasty crawfish dinner. The Forest Motel was a huge improvement over the last two nights. In the morning, the grandmotherly desk clerk said, with a worried look, "I do hope you have a safe journey."

"I always ride as safely as I can."

She told me, "A nice young man stayed with us a few weeks ago. He had ridden his bike through many of the states and was headed west just like you. It is only ten miles to Jeanerette, but he was hit and killed by a speeding car before he got there. I really worry about you."

With those reminders of my precarious lifestyle ringing in my ears, I pedaled toward Jeanerette.

Only forty-nine miles today as I wandered from U.S. 90 to State Highway 182 while checking access roads and nearby county roads in an unsuccessful search for a smooth surface and safe shoulder. Good news was that I not only made it to Jeanerette alive but had only the usual close calls with passing vehicles.

Further good news came when I stopped at a state patrol office to call a photo shop about my ailing camera. The shop was six miles off the highway and it was getting late. The patrol captain, hearing my end of the conversation, told one of his patrolmen to take me to the shop in his patrol car. While we waited for the camera to be repaired, the patrolman told of potential dangers that lay ahead for a lone bicyclist. After bringing me back to the state patrol office, he wished me safe traveling and I pedaled without incident to a Howard Johnson's before dark.

When I checked out the next morning, the desk clerk advised me to ride swiftly when I got to Lafayette as it was a "rough, tough neighborhood."

Although I hadn't let such warnings scare me, caution must have been on my mind as I rode into Lafayette at daybreak. At one intersection, a service station had not yet opened. Nearby, a group of young black men congregated around an empty phone booth. One man was urinating in the gutter. The light turned red. I stopped. He stared at me so I said, "Good morning."

"Mornin'," he muttered.

Another black man had been watching from across the street. He stepped off the curb and slowly edged toward me. It took forever for the light to change. When it did, I rode "swiftly," until I passed the sign "Leaving Lafayette, Louisiana."

Actually, there was never any evidence of danger or acts of hostility. No doubt overstimulated imagination, not reality, caused my uneasiness.

Traffic was moderate, drivers considerate. One fellow gave me a cheery beep. I waved. He was watching his rearview mirror and waved in return. The natives were friendly after all.

🚲 🚲 🚲

A sign: "Rayne City Chamber of Commerce welcomes you to Rayne, Frog Capital of the World." Chambers of commerce brag about the darnedest things!

Fifty miles east of Lake Charles, I found the most dog-friendly rest area of the trip. A sign proclaimed, "Pet Rest Area." From the sign, a path led to and around the base of a fire hydrant.

My clean and comfortable room in Lake Charles was at Motel 6. One thing I had learned on my trip is that if a place to camp was not available, an economical and reliable option was a Motel 6. They were somewhat spartan, but had comfortable beds, were invariably clean, and I always knew what services and facilities to expect. One problem: Motel 6s were infrequent along the secondary roads I often traveled.

I made up for the austerity of my motel room by dining at Paw Paw's Famous Boatside French Restaurant, The Pride of Lake Charles. While devouring bayou-style frog legs and drinking a glass of Blue Nun, I reflected on stories my dad told of his parents hooking a mule team to a wagon for their monthly trip to shop at the general store in Lake Charles. In the 1890s they lived on a plantation across the Calcasieu River from town and had to ford the sometimes dangerously high river to get essential supplies.

When I rode through in 1985, Lake Charles was the largest city in southwest Louisiana. Its high-rise skyline featured splendid hotels and magnificent restaurants. I stopped to photograph the Downtowner and Hilton Hotels, Calcasieu Marine Bank, Civic Center, and First Federal Building. As I photographed the Magnolia Life Building, an ultralight with pontoons flew a scarce 100 feet above my head. What would dad have thought of all that? I wondered.

🚲 🚲 🚲

At first light I was on the bike, cautiously working my way back to I-10. Just before I reached the Calcasieu River bridge on the freeway, a state patrol car passed and stopped on the shoulder ahead. A handsome young patrolman walked back and started wagging his finger under my nose as if I were a naughty boy. "That's a no-no. You can't ride that thing on the interstate," he smiled patronizingly.

I had checked bicycle regulations throughout this journey. All stated that unless reasonable alternatives were available or "Bicycles Prohibited" signs were present, one could ride on the interstate.

I patiently explained this to the young patrolman. He just as patiently listened, then issued his ultimatum. "Well, you can't ride on interstates in Louisiana."

"How do you propose I get to Texas?" I asked.

With apparent sincerity, he responded, "You just push your bike over that bridge, then push it to the Texas line."

"You have to be kidding! Isn't that about thirty miles away?"

"No, I'm not. Yes, it is," he said as he turned, walked back, and sat in the patrol car, watching me. I glumly began pushing toward the bridge.

Pushing the bike a mile and a half on a thirty-inch sidewalk high above the roadway required concentration, especially when the bridge shook violently as big trucks rolled past. If Old Faithful and I had fallen into traffic, we'd have looked worse than a road-killed 'possum.

Leaving the bridge, I looked back. The patrol car was out of sight. I jumped on the bike and pedaled west. Before reaching the Sabine River, which separates Louisiana from Texas, I stopped at a convenience store and told the clerk my sad story.

"Dozens of cyclists tell me the same thing," she said. "You shouldn't have any more trouble. Lots of eastbound cyclists stop here and tell of riding for miles on I-10 in Texas. That patrol guy in Lake Charles sure has his facts wrong."

I rode on. Texas was only five miles down the road.

To while away the twenty minutes to Texas, I pondered the societal implications of events along the last thousand miles or so of my journey. It seemed that almost daily—indeed, sometimes several times a day—local folks expressed distrust, not only of strangers, but of neighbors in the next town—or down the road a piece. What was going on? How could one live a fulfilled life with such anxieties about some kind of danger, violence, or other evil lurking just around the corner?

Carol and I, in the 1970s, had belonged to a faith community within our church. We spent many evenings talking about the lack of community within so-called communities. At the time, I was reading books by M. Scott Peck, M.D., that discussed psychology and religion. He was concerned, I recall, that so few had ever experienced true community, or even had a vision of it.

Peck contended that people do not like to accept bad news about themselves but are quite willing believe it about others, even neighbors. Could such a view be triggering the fearful anticipation of danger I have been routinely encountering? I'll ponder these things as I pedal west. Perhaps I can figure it out by the time I get across Texas. It's a big state.

CHAPTER THIRTEEN

Texas

The sun is riz.
The sun is set.
And we ain't out of Texas yet!

A huge sign in the middle of the Sabine River bridge proclaimed "Welcome to Texas. Drive Friendly, the Texas Way."

After I had enjoyed a wide, smooth shoulder for the first seven Texas miles, a car passed, pulled onto the shoulder ahead, and stopped. A man walked back with a smile and outstretched hand. "Howdy, where you heading with that good-looking bike?" After my explanation, he continued, "Name's Ray Post. Live up the road about fifteen miles. Come by my house, and you got your supper and a place to sleep tonight. We'll invite some folks over who enjoy cycling."

An hour later I met Ray again. He had driven home, hopped on his bike, and rode back five miles to make sure I didn't pass the turn to his house. We biked along picturesque back roads to his rural home where I met his wife, Shirley, and two grown sons, Dave and Jay.

Two neighbors came for dinner: Mikki, an enthusiastic cyclist, and Sheldon, who had planned a bicycle journey to visit all fifty states. After a start publicized by local newspapers and radio, he rode in eleven states before becoming ill and abandoning the trip. Ray said later that he thought Sheldon couldn't stand the loneliness. Ray hoped he would try again. I hoped so too, but never heard if he did.

Before dinner, we joined hands in the kitchen where Dave, a physical education teacher at the local middle school, prayed an eloquent grace thanking the Lord for guiding me to their home. Actually, Ray had helped the Lord out.

Dinner was a shrimp, chicken, and oyster gumbo; two terrific salads; and an assortment of desserts. All on short notice.

Ray and Shirley had begun bicycling the previous year. Each had already biked more than 100 miles in a day. Ray worked in an oil refinery for Texaco, but the oil boom was slacking off and the company had reduced its workforce drastically. When I met him, he was looking forward to retiring in three years at age fifty-five; then he and Shirley were planning some serious cycling.

Early the next morning, Shirley prepared a big country-style breakfast before I headed back to U.S. 90 and on toward Liberty.

As the day progressed, I had reason to question the meaning of the sign that admonished "Drive Friendly, the Texas Way." Several times before reaching Liberty, I heard a car accelerating directly behind me. A check of the rearview mirror would reveal a car roaring down *my* shoulder. The driver would then pull back into traffic and give me a dirty look while passing.

I asked the attendant at a service station what was going on. "Well," he said, "shoulders can be dangerous. When an impatient driver can't get past, he'll just pull out on the shoulder and pass on the right side. I don't think it's really legal, but here in Texas they do things different." They sure as hell do!

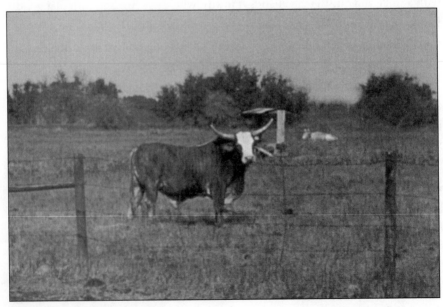

A Texas steer poses for his photo.

A few miles west of Liberty, I left U.S. 90 and took State Highway 321 to Cleveland where a couple of bearded natives cleared up something that had puzzled me since I noticed the town Cut and Shoot on a Texas map. Something was familiar about that name. It was, they told me, the home of Roy Harris, a heavyweight contender who fought in the 1940s. That was all I needed to remember hearing his fights on the radio. They said Harris still lived there. Later, folks in the Cut and Shoot Mercantile pointed out his large home and said he had a real estate business and was the county clerk.

I went to a library and checked in *King of the World* by David Remnick. This noted sportswriter, in writing about heavyweight fighters Floyd Patterson and Sonny Liston, had this to say:

> *Perhaps the most notable of Patterson's opponents before Liston was one Roy Harris of Cut and Shoot, Texas. As the papers were happy to point out, Harris grew up wrestling alligators in a swamp around his house known as the Big Thicket. He also was kin to an Uncle Clem and cousins Hominy, Coon, and Armadillo. In short, Harris was a PR setup, and still it took Floyd thirteen rounds to end it. Liston destroyed Harris in one.*

A friendly fellow in the mercantile explained how Cut and Shoot, population 568, got its name. Early in its history, there was a Baptist church at each end of town and, according to his story, "Ever' time the two churches got together for a picnic or a meetin', there would be a cuttin' or a shootin'—or both." I have never found documentation for the name's origin, but these Texans do have colorful stories.

On December 23 I reached the LaQuinta Motel in Houston to find the tall, lean manager carrying hand weights and walking briskly around the building. He told about his recovery from open-heart surgery in August and how great he felt after beginning a program of vigorous exercise.

After surveying road-weary Old Faithful and listening to an abbreviated story of my journey, he boomed, "You bet we have a place for you and your bike. First, let me store your bike in a room where it can stay over the holidays." He reinforced my belief that a healthy attitude about one's body leads to positive attitudes toward others and life in general.

Next day I flew from Houston to my son and daughter-in-law's Atlanta home for Christmas. It was special to be with family and later, to fly to East Lansing for New Year's Eve and a few days with Elisabeth.

Returning to Houston from my thirteen-day holiday break, I was enthusiastic to be on the last leg of my journey. San Diego was only 2,250 miles away.

The second morning after leaving Houston, I crossed the Brazos River in dense fog and was soon soaking wet from sweat and the fog. Water dripped off the rim of my helmet. Nine miles later I turned south on State Highway 36 until County Road 442 took me southwest across the San Bernard River to the tiny town of Boling, "Home of the Fighting Bulldogs, the 1972 AA football champions." Never mind that they hadn't won a championship in the fourteen years since. I love small-town pride.

🚲 🚲 🚲

Staying three nights in the Cattleman's Motel in Bay City wasn't on my itinerary, but preset agendas aren't always a reliable measure of the best thing to do. I had pedaled slowly into town, facing a cold headwind and spitting rain. It was raining next morning when the phone rang. Brian Lee, a reporter with the *Bay City Daily Tribune,* said the motel desk clerk had called to say that a cross-country cyclist was in town and she thought he might have an interesting story. I hadn't yet agreed to an interview and still felt the journey was too personal to share widely. But Brian's pleasant persistence won out. I was glad it did. First, I enjoyed the interview. Second, he took me to a fine restaurant in Bay City for dinner.

A bundle of unanswered letters demanded attention, and some business matters required typing. I called Spoonemore's Office Supply to check on a typewriter to rent. Manager Dan Ratliff said, "Come down and do your typing here."

At the busy store, I decided little serious work would be accomplished there. Although Office Supply didn't rent equipment, Dan offered, "For someone on a trip like yours, I'll put the best used typewriter we have in my van and bring it to your motel. Be out right away so you can get busy."

A few minutes after I had biked back to the motel room and closed the door, I heard, "Dwight, are you in there?"

Dan was standing outside with a heavy IBM Selectric II in his arms. Although he wanted me to get my work done, Dan sat on the bed, asking about my adventure and telling me highlights of his interesting life.

He was a fifty-five-year-old musician in addition to owning and managing his business. In his youth Dan had traveled with a band that played gigs in many places around the United States. He still had a four-piece band and was booked up during all his spare time. He lived on an offshore island. I invited Dan and his wife to go to dinner with me.

"I'd love to," he said, "but my wife has prepared a special dinner and a basket with wine and cheese for a drive out to our coastal home. At my stage of life, when your wife gets you fixed up with all that, you'd better take advantage of the romantic occasion." Thinking of similar times with Carol, I wistfully agreed.

🚲 🚲 🚲

Southwest of Blessing, on Farm Road 1862, the landscape changed from black agricultural soils to rough brushland. Several coveys of mourning doves flew from brush on either side of the highway. One white-winged dove displayed its large white wing patches and white tail corners as it zoomed across the highway scant yards ahead of me. Five miles later about fifteen scaled quail flashed their gaudy plumage as they decided the brush was greener on the other side of the road. Flashing is a good term to describe their light-colored feathers with dark-colored margins that look like iridescent fish scales. And seeing them in the air was a pleasant surprise, for they much prefer running.

Pastureland began to replace the mesquite and other shrubs. Herds of Black Angus and Herefords grazed where longhorn cattle once provided meat, hides, and horns, and inspired songs and stories, mostly exaggerated, about trail rides, shoot-outs, and failed cowboy romances.

At Sand Dollar Motel in Fulton, David Blankenship and his wife, Glenda, picked me up. Dave was the Audubon biologist headquartered in nearby Rockport. I knew him as a graduate student at Colorado State University.

Dave was scheduled for a Saturday evening talk about brown pelicans and whooping cranes. We took a ferry across Aransas Bay to Port Aransas where Dave gave an illustrated lecture in the auditorium of a University of Texas building to an audience of Sierra Club and Audubon Society members. His polished presentation gave me the warm glow of pride I always felt when one of our students had "done good."

An early morning "whooping crane tour" with Captain Ted Appell in his thirty-foot Pearson Cruiser was a glorious celebration of both the sabbath and creation. I photographed a sunrise, brown pelicans, double-crested cormorants, American oystercatchers, roseate spoonbills, and many others, but managed only one distant photo of three whooping cranes, the archetype of endangered species.

🚲　🚲　🚲

Rockport post office was one of the sixteen addresses around the United States where I had arranged to pick up general delivery mail. After church I was grousing to the motel clerk about having all of Sunday afternoon to read and respond to mail but wouldn't be able to pick it up until Monday morning. She smiled, "Pat Tedder, the postmaster over in Rockport, is a real accommodating guy. You could call his home. Maybe he can figure something out."

I wasn't optimistic but called anyway. He was outside preparing a barbeque dinner. Lamely, I explained my problem to his wife and ended with, "This is a bad time to call. I'll see him tomorrow morning in the post office."

"Oh, no," she replied, "he'll want to talk with you." He did and quickly came up with a strategy.

"I'll put the ribs and chicken on the grill and someone can watch them. Then I'll drive to the post office, pick up your mail, and bring it to your motel." My offer to bike the five miles and meet him at the post office fell on deaf ears. "You just stay put at the Sand Dollar. I'll be there in a half hour."

Right on time Pat drove up with a bundle of mail and a big grin. He waved aside my thanks and offer to pay him for his trouble with, "Boy, that sounds like a great ride you're taking. Get your packages ready and come by in the morning. Well, gotta go before they eat up all the chicken and ribs."

I couldn't believe it. Even for Small Town, America, this was extravagant generosity.

The post office was closed next morning when I arrived with letters and two packages to mail, but someone was noisily working inside the small building. Responding to my shouts, Pat came to the door.

"Well, you're bright and early. We're not open, but give me your packages and we'll get you on your way." With that, Pat weighed the packages, took my $3.14, and told me the best route to Sinton where I would visit the Welder Wildlife Refuge.

  

James Teer, director of the refuge, met me at the gate and escorted me to a room in their dormitory. Jim and I had known each other only through our scientific publications, but I couldn't have asked for a warmer welcome. After getting settled, I rode quietly around the largest private refuge in the world to observe and photograph the wildlife. It was beautiful and peaceful. I saw twenty white-tailed deer and a multitude of waterfowl and shorebirds, listened to coyote serenades, and photographed a large V of Canada geese silhouetted against an exquisite sunset. A luminous harvest moon begged to become part of my memories, so I took its picture, too. I was enjoying riding in the moonlight, so there was no need to hurry.

  

Leaving Motel 6 in Kingsville, I rode to the King Ranch. The owners had recognized the value of wildlife and after a century of emphasizing cattle and horses, hired Bill Kiel, a professional biologist, to manage these resources. Bill told me that the ranch once covered 1.25 million acres but had now been reduced to four divisions with a total of 825,000 acres. That is nearly 1,300 square miles. Still quite a spread.

Six years before they had begun leasing hunting rights on 82,000 acres. Sportsmen clubs or partnerships held three-year leases, with options to renew for additional three-year periods. That gave hunters a long-term interest in the management of wildlife. About 25,000 northern bobwhites and 1,500 white-tailed deer were harvested each year. In addition, javelina and a multitude of waterfowl species were hunted on the ranch. They also cultivated 35,000 acres for crops such as sorghum and cotton.

 &#xfe de; 

In Freer, population 3,213, I pitched my tent near the Ford garage where they let me use the employee shower. After dinner at a twenty-four-hour restaurant, I was in the sack by 7:20 P.M.

Morning came early. At 2:45 A.M. raindrops began hitting the tent. The sky looked threatening so I performed some perfunctory exercises inside the tent, used the garage bathroom they had left open for me, and packed Old Faithful in the faint rays of a distant streetlight. By 4:30 A.M. I was back at the all-night restaurant.

The waitress told me it was seventy miles to Cotulla with no towns and only a few ranches along the way. To prepare for this, I asked her to make a sandwich while I ate breakfast. She then filled my three bottles with ice water while I went outside and pumped the tires. At a nearby convenience store, I stocked up with an apple, orange, banana, trail mix, and a couple of candy bars.

After I had traveled eighteen miles north on U.S. 16, serious rain began. I tied a tiny plastic bag over the odometer, a larger bag over the front pannier to protect the tape recorder and camera, and a trash can liner over my sleeping bag and other gear lashed over the back panniers. It was still dark.

In pilot training I was told not to fly into clouds, storms, or any conditions when the horizon was not visible. In those circumstances, unless the pilot focused entirely on the instrument panel, he might become dizzy and confused, a condition called "vertigo." I always nodded politely, but wondered if it was a lot of baloney. This morning I found it was not.

When the white line defining the shoulder was even faintly visible, I could maintain control. But in repaired or other areas without the line, I would immediately start "losing it." Panic would set in. Was I about to go off the right side of the highway? Or was I drifting over the left embankment? I couldn't even tell if the bike was moving. Sometimes, when totally confused, I would squeeze the brake levers, feel like the bike was tipping over, lean to the side and put my foot down, only to find, with one heck of a jerk, that I was still moving.

I could have stopped, of course. But it *was* sort of fascinating.

In early dawn light I coasted into the Nueces River basin. Five golden eagles, a couple of red-tailed hawks, three northern harriers, a few horned larks, and some killdeers enlivened the basin crossing.

Riding the first thirty-six miles toward Cotulla on Ranch Road 624, I had counted nine mailboxes but saw only four sets of ranch buildings. As the waitress in Freer had foretold, it sure was lonely country.

Nearer Cotulla, population 3,912, there were oil wells, agricultural lands, and more farm and ranch buildings. A large sign proclaimed "Myers Memorial Stadium." The high school football field boasted banks of lights for night games and stands that would hold several thousand fans. I remembered Freer, with its lighted tennis courts and covered stands for spectators. These small towns in Texas were great supporters of their athletes.

In a tiny restaurant at Big Wells, population 939, a young waitress with captivating Spanish brown eyes showed again that small-town Texans have big hearts. I ordered a cup of coffee and asked if they had a sweet roll or doughnut to go with it. They didn't. But the waitress said, "There is a grocery store nearby. I'll get something there." When I protested, she insisted, "It's only a block away. I'll hurry and be right back." In a few minutes she came in, out of breath after running all the way down and back to get a chocolate cake. She cut a huge piece, and I left a large tip.

As I was getting on my bike outside the restaurant, a fellow came out with his young daughter and said, "You must be traveling a long ways."

"How did you know?"

"I saw you riding over near Freer. That's a hundred miles from here."

This was just one of several recent instances when small-town or rural folks let me know they were keeping tabs on me. I wanted to wander the back roads of America forever!

This enthusiasm didn't last long. Two days earlier I had biked seventy miles and felt fine. Yesterday, after only fifty-one miles, my entire body ached. I was exhausted. Last night, I had awakened at 12:30 A.M. with cold feet and my face feeling on fire. There wasn't much sleep after that. I recalled similar sensations ignored too long last year in South Carolina.

A peek outside at 5:30 A.M. revealed a dreary scene of dense fog. This, plus nausea and a splitting headache, told me it wasn't going to be a good day. After a light breakfast, I forced myself onto the bike and pedaled cautiously into dense fog, headed for Uvalde where a former graduate student, Dwight Guynn, was expecting me.

Twenty-two miles of headache, nausea, and fatigue later, I began to vomit and consider the possibility of delaying completion of this journey once again. That thought hurt more than my body.

I must have looked as bad as I felt when Dwight opened his door to greet me. I blurted that I didn't feel well but nothing was seriously wrong. Dwight said, "Sit down. I'll get you a glass of water and call my doctor."

In a few minutes he reported, "It's Sunday, but Dr. Smythe says to bring you over to his house and he'll have a look at you."

My temperature was 104 degrees and, from my complaints of low back pain and bloody and painful urination, Dr. Smythe's tentative diagnosis was prostatitis. He stated flatly, "You are in no condition to be riding your bike. I urge you to return home to your own doctors for more thorough evaluation and treatment. You can decide if you want to finish your trip after you recuperate."

ᘓᗝ ᘓᗝ ᘓᗝ

I left Old Faithful with the Guynns and flew back to Fort Collins where my urologist described the problem as "urinary tract infection with significant prostatic enlargement" and prescribed the antibiotic Bactrim to be taken for six weeks. "After that," he concluded, "you may be able to return to your bike tour, but you must understand that biking is not good for your prostate, so you may have more trouble."

I understood. But there were only 1,800 more miles of biking left, and I wasn't going to stop because of my damn prostate.

ᘓᗝ ᘓᗝ ᘓᗝ

At 8:30 P.M. on February 10, 1986, Dwight met me at the Uvalde bus station after I had flown back from Fort Collins. I had been off the ride for twenty-three days. Getting over the infection and ready to ride again had taken less time than the doctor predicted but much longer than I wanted.

The next morning we drove to the Corazon Ranch where Dwight introduced me to the owner, "Doc" Belcher, a retired veterinarian. When Doc took over Corazon Ranch, a regular livestock ranching operation had been underway for many years. A new objective for Belcher, a well-trained geneticist, was to import wildlife from around the world and strengthen their bloodlines or create new varieties.

I admired Doc Belcher's skill in developing sturdy animals adapted to the harsh Texas environment. I only wished he had stayed with raising livestock. Imported wildlife, even if genetically "improved," too often have increased to the detriment of native species and their habitat.

武 武 武

A wild taxi ride took me from Del Rio, Texas, over the Rio Grande to Ciudad Acuna, Mexico. After a dinner of *pescado en salsa blanca,* meaning "lake bass cooked in white sauce," I shopped for a wedding gift for Elisabeth's son and his fiancée. Although one is expected to wrangle over prices in Mexico, I hate to barter. My first offer of a few pesos less than the asking price was met by a smaller drop in price. I quickly paid and the sidewalk merchant seemed disappointed that our transaction ended so abruptly.

Before heading out of Del Rio the next morning, I stopped to photograph a sign that proclaimed "Jesus Is Coming Very Soon!"

Directly behind the sign was Del Rio Monument Company, which advertised tombstones for sale. Was there some humorous irony in this, or was I getting a little weird?

Ten miles west of Del Rio, the United States and Mexico had constructed Armistad Reservoir during the 1965–69 period. Now, it was operated under supervision of the International Boundary and Water Commission. The dam impounded waters of the Rio Grande, Pecos, and Devils Rivers. One of the largest reservoirs in the United States, Armistad had 800 miles of rugged shoreline.

Biking along the reservoir's edge, I was amazed by the fancy restaurants, lodges, motels, and saloons. Several RV parks, containing hundreds of motor homes and campers, extended from near the shoreline out into the surrounding barren shrublands.

武 武 武

"Langtry, Texas. Home of the Late Judge Roy Bean, the West's Most Colorful and Controversial Justice of the Peace" read the sign.

I rushed to the post office to mail film, tapes, and letters before it closed at noon. And since it had been over twenty-four hours since my last hot meal,

I sprinted over to Bud and Patsy's, more bar than restaurant, but the only place in Langtry that served food. I asked if I could still get breakfast.

"We're fixin' us a breakfast," said Bud. "We'll just add a little more for you."

I didn't ask what was on the menu but Patsy offered, "We call it breakfast tacos in this country." Whatever its name, the flour tortillas, eggs, hash browns, and a strong-flavored but tasty meat disappeared quickly.

When I had finished, she said, "You've been eating illegal wild venison. We can't charge for it, but we'll accept a donation." Glad to leave a generous tip, I drank a final cup of coffee and wondered if I had been introduced to Judge Bean's famous "Law West of the Pecos."

The well-publicized Judge Roy Bean Visitor Center didn't impress me. The dioramas with sound and music told exaggerated tales about the old frontier justice of the peace, also called "the hangin' judge."

More restrained historians claim the closest Judge Bean ever came to sentencing a man to hanging was to bang the gavel on the bar top in the Jersey Lilly Saloon where he held court and proclaimed, "I'm finin' you your gun, a round of drinks for the jury, and ever' cent in your pocket. If you show up in Langtry again, you'll be wearing a noose for a necktie. Case dismissed." Then the judge would put his toweling apron on and go back to tending bar.

At least that's the legend.

A story in the February 1984 *National Geographic* stated that Roy Bean had promoted the Maher-Fitzsimmons world heavyweight boxing championship fight in 1896 thereby putting Langtry on the map. Jack Skiles, supervisor of the Roy Bean Visitor Center, said, according to that article, "When all those eastern sportswriters got out here, they didn't have much copy. The old judge put on a show for them, and they made him famous."

After checking into a motel on U.S. 90 a short distance out of Langtry, I hiked along the bluffs overlooking the Rio Grande to get a feel for the country. In the evening I returned to Bud and Patsy's for dinner.

Most of the time a couple of men played pool on the one pool table. Most conversations centered on ranching operations, neighbors and their kids, fishing, and, of course, tall tales of drinking and carousing. I didn't hear anyone talk about hunting, but there was much interest in guns and shooting at all kinds of targets.

One fellow who had been in the bar at noon asked me, "What ya been doin' all afternoon?"

"Hiked down toward the river and photographed some beaver ponds in a creek that comes into the Rio Grande."

A heavy woman, also in the bar at noon, was still there. She spoke up. "Yeah, we used to go down and shoot those sonsabitches."

This reminded a fellow of fishing the Rio Grande between Comstock and Langtry. "We usta take a picnic basket and cooler full of beer in the boat. When we threw an empty bottle in the river, we'd shoot at it 'til we sunk the damn thing."

One fellow glanced at me before saying, "That's so them environmental fellers won't say we're litterin' the ol' river." Nothing was said about catching fish.

"Varmints," mostly badgers, was the next topic. "Those mean ol' critters. If they run outta roots an' stuff, they'll kill a goat. I once't saw a badger chew the head off a goat with them powerful jaws an' big ol' teeth. They oughta kill alla them."

Another chimed in with stories of eagles killing lambs. "Them damn birds ain't good for nuthin 'but shootin'."

Finally I said, "You guys sure shoot a helluva lot of things around here."

An old sheepman sitting at the bar pulled himself up, turned toward me, and said, "If it ain't a goat, if it ain't a sheep, if it ain't human, it don't belong and we shoot the sonofabitch!"

The population of Langtry was forty-five. Most in the bar were from surrounding ranches. I heard one rancher say it took him an hour to get to town; another said he lived two hours away.

Conversation flowed easily among neighbors and old friends. Honest concern for one another's welfare was evident. As several prepared for the long drive home, they weren't "staggerin' drunk," but some wouldn't have passed a sobriety test either. Those with a long way to go began leaving before nine o'clock. A favorite departure routine featured a bear hug for the lady, a vigorous handshake or back slap for the man, and the admonition, "You drive careful now, y'hear."

Their attitudes about law enforcement, environment, wildlife, and education differed vastly from mine; but these were down-to-earth, caring, generous folks. Still, a dead eagle is a dead eagle!

ڵ   ڵ   ڵ

The warm sun felt good on my back. Two sets of stretching exercises before leaving Langtry lessened the lower back pain that had plagued me off and on since Uvalde.

After ten miles I was hurting again. I lay on a picnic table while completing another set of stretching exercises. That would get me a few more miles.

Another fifteen miles of rough highway, strong headwinds, and I stopped for an energy bar and stretched out on the roadside with my helmet for a pillow but the pain didn't allow me to relax.

Finally, I reached Dryden. Over three hours to ride the last thirteen miles. Only thirty-nine miles all day.

Bill, postmaster and proprietor of Dryden Mercantile, sold me nine dollars' worth of groceries and offered, "You're welcome to pitch your tent back of the store." He left for Sanderson after letting me fill my empty water bottles. I used one to pour water over my hands, face, and feet; then wiped them off before turning in early. I relaxed and slept soundly until 5:45 A.M.

Striking camp quickly, I walked the empty streets past boarded up buildings as doors banged in the wind. If tumbleweeds had rolled down the dusty street, I would have sworn it was a western movie set.

Bill returned at 7:00 A.M. and assured me that, though I hadn't seen a soul, six people did live in Dryden. Then he set about making coffee in the back of the store and visited as I had V8 juice, two cups of coffee, and an apple cinnamon roll heated in the microwave. Thus fortified, I set out.

High, gusting wind, a steady climb, and a constantly paining back led me to "tough it out" only twenty-five miles before stopping in Sanderson, wondering how long it would take to get to San Diego.

The following morning, four miles out of Sanderson, a ferocious gust of wind tore Old Faithful from my grasp and we went down together. Attempting to record the event, I found the toggle switch controlling the tape recorder had broken off in the fall. Now I would have to dig the recorder out of the handlebar bag every time I wanted to tape events as they happened.

By midafternoon I had traveled only twenty-six miles and the last nine had taken more than two hours. Fighting gusting, twisting headwinds had painfully strained my left hip and hamstring. I was totally exhausted and at least thirty miles from Marathon, the next town. No cars had passed me for two hours.

I sat down and began to assess the situation. Obviously, I wasn't going to reach a campground or motel by nightfall. By pedaling slowly and walking when necessary, I reasoned, I could find a spot sheltered from the wind. My tent and sleeping bag would protect me from the elements overnight. Two of my three water bottles were still full. An apple, orange, and can of V8 juice would ease my thirst. The panniers held trail mix, dried fruit, energy bars, and crackers with peanut butter and cheese.

Even if back pain and the headwinds continued, I might make it to Marathon tomorrow. If not, I could survive a second night in the tent and finish the following day.

A red pickup went past, stopped, turned around, and came back. The driver, a man about thirty, got out and said, "It must be awfully tough to ride into this headwind. Can I give you a ride?" My benefactor was Irvin Cox. He lived on a nearby ranch and was headed for Marathon.

I felt chagrined, however, at accepting a ride. In the past I had "cheated" only twice on my resolve to pedal every mile of the way. Once, a construction employee took me across a few miles of newly laid asphalt. The second time was when I reached the Golden Gate Bridge where I found the bridge was closed to bicyclists, but the highway department provided a van and trailer to periodically haul cyclists and their bicycles across. But this was the first time I had conceded to fatigue or pain—and that hurt.

One advantage of being plain tuckered out was that I kept my big mouth shut and instead of asking a lot of questions, just listened.

Irvin's family had once owned a huge ranch. Eventually, they divided it into three ranches. His parents operated one, a brother and his family another, and Irvin lived with an eighty-eight-year-old aunt on the third ranch, which he managed. It was very boring out on the ranch, he said, so he was driving to town to see if there was any "action."

At the Gage Hotel in Marathon, I thanked him for giving me a much-needed lift and wished him well in whatever lay ahead.

The half-hour reprieve from battling the wind did wonders. After registering at the Hotel, I biked to the other end of town, had coffee, then conducted a self-guided tour. The Catholic church was open so I went in to kneel and pray for my family and for strength and perseverance.

🚲 🚲 🚲

Alpine, Texas, is described as "a sparkling little city nestled nearly a mile high in the Davis Mountains."

After a night in a dormitory on Sul Ross State University campus, I biked to Alpine airport before sunrise and rented a Cessna 150. Early morning sunlight cast shadows across the rugged volcano-formed peaks of the Davis Mountains as I flew north over Fort Davis and climbed above ponderosa pine forests to circle the world-renowned McDonald Observatory.

Enchanted by this scenic area, I entertained ideas of spending a few years here after the bike trip. But there were important considerations. While crossing the southern tier of states toward the finish line, my thoughts often turned to ideas about sharing the rest of my life with Elisabeth. But, at this point, there were many unknowns. Elisabeth's impeccable home in East Lansing and her long tenure as executive secretary for the president of the Coca-Cola Division headquartered in Lansing would be hard for her to leave.

Nevertheless, the clear, unpolluted air and scenic beauty inspired me to dream while sliding smoothly over the descending landscape from the Davis Mountains to land on the airfield just outside town.

I reluctantly put aside my dreams and got underway on my bike a little after 10:00 A.M. Seven hours later I had pedaled only thirty-seven miles along State Highway 118 from Alpine to Davis Mountain State Park. This lack of progress happily resulted from numerous stops to photograph herds of pronghorn and cattle on lush grasslands, and attractive ranches nestling in green valleys backed by pine-covered hills.

After dinner at Indian Lodge, I pitched my tent among the Emory oak, one-seed juniper, and fragrant sumac along Keesey Creek. The four-syllable hoo-hoo-hoo-hoo of a white-winged dove and softer ooah-oo-oo-oo of a mourning dove quickly lulled me to sleep. Soon, rattling of something invading the panniers on my bicycle roused me. Forgetting flashlight and glasses, I unzipped the tent and let fly with a rock at a dimly seen animal bounding across the dry creek bed. Not fully awake, I staggered back into the tent and snuggled back into the sleeping bag.

The rattling started again. This time the flashlight's beam revealed two raccoons scurrying away. The only way to dissuade these mischievous scamps was to remove temptation, so I moved the panniers into the tent and then slept soundly until awakened by an early morning duet of the doves.

While eating breakfast I read about Fort Davis, where I planned to spend the next night. The site was selected in 1854 in response to depredations on settlers and travelers of the San Antonio–El Paso Trail by Apaches, Kiowas, and Comanches. Named after Jefferson Davis, U.S. secretary of war and later president of the southern Confederacy, Fort Davis was one of the first posts to receive black soldiers. They compiled such a record as fierce fighters that their Apache and Comanche antagonists, in respect, called them "buffalo soldiers."

I saw a variety of wildlife while riding thirteen miles toward the McDonald Observatory. First a greater roadrunner, then a few pronghorn, and farther into the oak- and juniper-covered hills, scaled and Montezuma quail, many songbirds, and small herds of mule deer.

At the visitor center, I accepted the invitation of Curt Laughlin, supervisor of the observatory program, to ride the final steep mile to the observatory on the summit of 6,800-foot Mount Locke. The 200-ton dome I had photographed from the air two days earlier was even more impressive up close where I saw the 107-inch telescope inside.

                              🚲   🚲   🚲

Pedaling west on State Highway 166, I came around a curve and almost ran into five mule deer. There were several other groups of seven or fewer. Pronghorn were also abundant.

A handsome ranch house on a bluff overlooked thousands of acres of productive grassland. Rugged mountains stood all around. A large herd of cattle, mostly Herefords and white-faced Angus, grazed the vast landscape. Pronghorn foraged among them. Or stood, alert. Or bounded away, flared white-rump patches reflecting the morning sunlight in a dazzling display called a "heliograph." What diversity. What pastoral beauty.

Powder-puff clouds dotted an azure sky. The natural landscape, attractive ranches, and abundant wildlife formed a breathtaking scene. Even occasional hills and headwinds failed to discourage me. I arrived in Van Horn in disbelief that my longest day in weeks, 82.3 miles, had passed so pleasantly.

This upbeat mood continued into Sunday as I rushed off to a Spanish-language mass. It was the perfect way to begin the day, though I understood few words. The singing captivated me. The enthusiastic young priest's hands, facial expressions, and voice brought eloquence to unfamiliar words. Understanding the structure of mass, I was comfortable with the prayers and readings, and appreciated the reverence so evident throughout the service.

Reveling in the satisfaction of the previous day's ride, I enjoyed a leisurely breakfast. After emptying the panniers, checking condition and completeness of clothing and equipment, and repacking everything, I cleaned, adjusted, and lubricated the bike.

A late morning tour of Van Horn didn't take long, and I began itching to get on the road again. So I did. And enjoyed the thirty-seven miles to Sierra Blanca.

🚲 🚲 🚲

Next morning I was at the Chuckwagon Cafe on the west end of Sierra Blanca. Before the pretty Mexican waitress could take my order, another waitress charged out of the kitchen, past the tables, and out the front door. Soon, I heard a man's angry voice and saw him pacing back and forth in the kitchen as he reprimanded the remaining waitress who was working furiously to serve customers. Her distressed countenance would dissolve into a smile as she approached a table and took an order. Then she rushed back into the kitchen to listen to more abuse.

By this time, six tables had filled with tourists, another with five men who appeared to be local laborers. I was at a table alone. The harried waitress was becoming visibly upset, and I had become convinced that my expectation of a quick breakfast, or even any breakfast, was in jeopardy.

I jumped up and walked to the open kitchen door. A tall, lanky guy, cowboy hat cocked on the back of his head, chair leaned back, and cowboy boots propped on a small table, was drinking coffee. To make sure I was talking to the right person, I asked, "Are you the man having some personnel problems this morning?"

His chair banged down. He looked at me open-mouthed. Finally he blurted, "Yeah, I guess we got a little problem here."

"Well," I replied, "I've got a little problem, too. I came in expecting a quick breakfast. The way you're hassling this young lady, I don't see how she gets any work done at all."

The cafe full of people had been forced to listen to his ranting. Now there wasn't a sound in the place as they listened to us. Obviously, he hadn't planned on this. "Just close the door, come in, and sit down," he stammered.

"I don't have any idea what your problem is," I retorted. "I don't want to come in and sit down. I just want to have breakfast in peace and be on my way. If you don't back off, I don't think that's going to happen."

As I turned and walked back to my table, two of the laborers grinned and gave me a "thumbs up" signal. The woman seated in the booth behind me turned and said, "Thank you for doing that. My husband and I were wishing someone would say something."

When I paid my bill, the waitress still was on the run. She smiled and asked, "Was everything all right?"

"Because of you, it sure was," I answered, handing her a five-dollar bill after paying the breakfast tab.

"Oh, you shouldn't," she whispered as tears pooled in her brown eyes.

"From what I've seen this morning," I countered, "whatever tips you get are far less than you deserve."

"I'm just trying to do my job." The pools spilled over. I wanted to hug her. Instead, I grabbed my helmet and pedaled west on I-10.

I thought about the lady's remark that she and her husband wished someone would say something. That seems to apply to many of us who wait for "George" to speak up.

My thoughts shifted to my tough old lumberjack dad. His contempt for a man who was afraid to speak out against injustice was portrayed by his frank but indelicate reproach: "He wouldn't say shit if his mouth was full of it."

Dad would have been proud of me that morning.

A few miles west of Sierra Blanca, I-10 bent southward until it reached the Rio Grande. Three hundred and seventy miles had slipped beneath the wheels since I had abandoned the grand old river at Langtry to pursue a more northerly route. I turned onto Farm Road 192 and, again, the land seemed hard and inhospitable along the Rio Grande. Tiny communities with names like Esperanza and Tornillo signaled closeness to Mexico.

No single incident gave reason for concern, but unfamiliar communities caused me to feel uneasy. I stopped, hid wallet inside map case, stuck credit card in a pocket inside biking shorts, and began rehearsing strategies in case I ran into banditos. Then I felt foolish and unworthy for doing so.

Cotton bolls tangled along the road told of last year's harvest. A few fields were being prepared for new crops.

McNary consisted of seven businesses: museum, gift shop, grocery, two service stations, garage with sign "Mechanic On Duty," and what appeared to be a factory. All abandoned. Windows broken. Doors open. Accentuating the loneliness, a fierce wind began howling through the empty buildings and sweeping sand past mesquite and saltbush scattered among the sand dunes.

The same desolate landscape greeted me at Lovelady Park near Fort Hancock. A stone monument read "In Memory of Dan Lovelady, 1964." Cigarette butts and broken beer bottles surrounded it. Trash festooned adjacent bushes. A large pile of nearby garbage stank. Among all this a sign implored "Hear My Voice, Oh God." Not far away, another proclaimed "Jesus Is My Salvation."

Similar signs had abounded in the Bible Belt from the piney woods of Georgia, through Florida, Alabama, Mississippi, and Louisiana, to this hardscrabble land along the Rio Grande in west Texas. Righteous pronouncements surrounded by profane desecration of the Creator's works seem to emphasize "dominion" while ignoring the many scriptural references to "stewardship."

🚲 🚲 🚲

After the clean, invigorating air of the Davis Mountains, it was a shock to see sullen brown smog obscuring the hills ahead as I left Desert Air Motel in Fabens and headed toward El Paso.

It must have been early lunch break at the high school in Clint, population 1,314. Dozens of students streamed across a vacant lot to stores along the main drag. A group of six Mexican boys neared a convenience store as I rode in. Their attire included flashy, brilliantly colored shirts and baggy pants. A few had a chain swinging between front and back pocket. Their black hair was well-oiled and slicked straight back in a sort of ducktail. They reminded me of the zoot-suiters of the 1940s.

As I leaned my bike against the store's front window, they formed a semi-circle around me while staring intently at Old Faithful and her heavy load. "Hi, fellas," I greeted them. No one spoke. "Have to use the bathroom and get a few things in the store. Sure would appreciate it if you kept an eye on my bike." Not a word. Two or three shot surprised glances my way.

They had moved in a little closer, still eyeing the bike and talking in low tones when I came out ten minutes later. "Thanks, guys," I said while putting on gloves and helmet. "I have a lot of valuable stuff and would have worried if you hadn't watched it for me." The latter was bullshit, of course. But I had vowed at the outset of this journey that trust, not fear, would be my guiding principle no matter how foolhardy it seemed. I hadn't tested that theory enough lately. Now that I had, I wasn't sure what I had proved. They didn't appear menacing, just remained silent as they drifted back to school, glancing back toward me.

Before I got out of the parking lot, a sheriff's car with two Mexican deputies in it drove up. One asked where I was headed and whether I had been hassled. They were friendly and we chatted for a few minutes about my trip.

Both deputies were astounded I'd not had any troubles and were still warning me to be careful of "illegals and other unsavory characters in this country" as they drove on.

Later in Anthony, I paused at an intersection to consult my map. Two teenage Mexicans in work clothes walked over from a nearby car wrecking business. "Need some help, sir?" one asked.

"Trying to figure the best road for biking to Las Cruces," I responded.

"Well, sir," the other said, "if you take this road," and he traced a line with his grimy finger, "you'll go through a lot of pecan groves. The trees make it shady and there's not as much wind." After a thoughtful pause, he smiled and his voice softened. "It's not much further, sir, and it is so beautiful." A poet in greasy coveralls. I followed his advice.

ᗦᗩ ᗦᗩ ᗦᗩ

As I stood on the pedals to top a hill in El Paso, a sudden ticketa-ticketa-tic signaled a problem. After carrying 250 pounds of bike, gear, and me for 12,737 miles, a spoke had finally broken. Rubbing sweat off my nose,

I looked to the right. I had stopped precisely in front of the Bike Peddler Shop. Though it was near closing time, the manager promised to replace the spoke, check wheels and tires, perform the major tune-up I requested, and have the bike ready to pick up by eight o'clock the next morning. They must have worked long after closing hours, but it was ready in the morning, and I was on my way.

That morning I crossed the state line into New Mexico. A total of 1,304 miles had passed beneath Old Faithful's tires since we crossed the Sabine River into Texas. They were miles packed with mind-boggling contrasts of landscapes, people, and events.

It was quite a ride, pardner.

CHAPTER FOURTEEN

Southwestern Desert

There is something about the desert ... There is some-thing there which the mountains, no matter how grand and beautiful, lack; which the sea, no matter how shin-ing and vast and old, does not have. ... The desert is dif-ferent. ... The desert waits outside, desolate and still and strange. ... Even after years of intimate contact and search, this quality of strangeness in the desert remains undiminished. Transparent and intangible as sunlight, yet always and everywhere present, it lures a man on and on, from the red-walled canyons to the smoke-blue ranges beyond ...

—Edward Abbey,
Desert Solitaire

New Mexico, Land of Enchantment. How could I associate enchantment with the dusty, parched, and often-abandoned villages along Highway 85 between the Texas–New Mexico border and Las Cruces? But the names—Berino, Vado, La Mesa, San Miguel, Mesilla—evoked visions of the Spanish conquistadors who pushed into what is now New Mexico, mingled their blood with the native Indian to form La Raza, the New Breed, and in 1595 established the first in a line of gov-ernors who have served—under four flags—to the present. In 1610, a decade before the Pilgrims landed on Plymouth Rock, Santa Fe became the capital where the Palace of the Governors is the oldest public building in the United States.

Pedaling through canyons, across mesas, and past buttes while watching the sun's rays embrace their haunting beauty, I began to appreciate the term "enchantment." Gazing at the night sky from my sleeping bag while the desert worked its magic, I could agree with John Gunther who poetically described this land as, "the purple desert flowing endlessly under lonely stars."

From *Life on the Line* by Mark Kramer and Danny Lehman, I found that the Rio Grande, called Rio Bravo del Norte by our neighbors in Mexico, constitutes half of the ragged 1,950-mile border between the two countries. The Rio Grande is born in melting snowbanks at 12,000 feet along the Continental Divide in Colorado. Water droplets coalesce into tiny rivulets that join to become creeks. Creeks, guided by terrain features and gravity, ultimately merge as the Rio Grande.

Where terrain is steep, the fledgling river plunges through deep canyons, racing toward the far-off Gulf of Mexico. Before leaving Colorado the river calms, wandering as the valleys widen, and man has built dams and diversions to put the water to agricultural, industrial, and domestic uses.

Where my route first intercepted the river at Del Rio, Texas, the elevation is 950 feet above sea level. I had missed 400 miles of the lower Rio Grande. From Del Rio I had followed it upstream for sixty-seven miles through harsh shrublands to Langtry, where I abandoned the grand old river for a 340-mile northwesterly shortcut until rejoining it at Esperanza, still in Texas. The land became gentler, the valley wider, and I saw pecan orchards and fields of wheat and barley. Lettuce, onions, and other row crops were also abundant on irrigated land as I progressed across the state line into New Mexico, then continued along U.S. 85 to Hatch.

The bed at Hatch Motel was reasonably comfortable but the return of back pain was a troubling reminder of difficult days and nights while crossing Texas. I hoped this wasn't going to be, as Yogi Berra once said, "déjà vu all over again."

As I continued northward, the land appeared even more productive, homes more prosperous. Many small farms advertised "Chili for Sale." This meant "chili peppers" but here, I was told, they just say "chili."

Near Garfield, I passed a beautiful hacienda-style home with well-groomed grounds and a graceful stone and wrought iron fence in front. Chili peppers grew in large irrigated fields on either side.

State Highway 90 led me west by southwest from Caballo on toward the Pacific Ocean. San Diego and the end of my journey were less than 900 miles away.

As I climbed toward Hillsboro, elevation 5,180 feet, chili pepper fields gave way to ranches where Brangus and Charolais beef cattle grazed in lush pastures.

After settling in at the S Bar X Motel and Saloon in Hillsboro, I showered and walked down the street to the Black Range Museum to learn more about the community. The "Bonanza" claim, I found, paid out over $1 million during the winter of 1877–78, and one lone miner "enriched the stores and saloons with $90,000 in gold dust and nuggets that winter." Two years later there were four saloons, four grocery stores, and four companies of soldiers, along with 300 miners who formed a militia to protect the area from Indians resenting the takeover of their lands. Equally feared were the lawless, including the Kinney Gang, the Dalton Gang, Butch Cassidy, and Jesse James.

Entertainment was provided by "the world's most beautiful woman monte dealer, Lottie Deno, who parted the miners from their money in a gambling hall and saloon." Other amenities were the pleasures and services furnished by Madame Sadie, an émigré from the brothels of London's Limehouse district in 1886. She operated her own brothel as well as a restaurant and hotel, and a stagecoach and express that carried the riches from the mines to the railhead. Sadie was also an "angel of mercy" when the flu epidemic of 1918 caused death and panic in the village. Sadie and her "girls," it was reported, "cooked, fed the sick, cared for the orphans, and laid out the dead."

I pedaled out of Hillsboro's lusty history while the stars were still visible and a half moon glowed softly. It was good that I enjoyed the moment because, several times during the night I awoke with severe pain.

After the first five hours, mostly in the lowest gear and pedaling hard, I had traveled only 17.5 miles and climbed 3,048 feet to the top of 8,228-foot Emory Pass where I encountered the first snowbank since May 5 last year when I crossed Stevens Pass in the Cascades.

The afternoon featured a descent of 2,328 feet and a dozen stops to photograph the hill country of New Mexico before reaching Silver City. Pain persisted but muscle spasms decreased, and I was satisfied with sixty-six miles for the day.

Next morning I was ready for prayer and reflection at Saint Francis Newman Church. Father Bryant had noticed my bicycle locked in front of the church. Seeing me stuff my helmet under the pew, he stepped down from the altar and delayed mass while welcoming me to the community.

I thoroughly enjoyed his down-to-earth message. An excellent guitarist accompanied the mostly-Spanish singing. My sagging spirits soared until I knelt. That's when back spasms hit again. I wiggled, squirmed, and wobbled my butt back and forth, up and down, trying to stop the pain. Sweat poured from my temples. Finally my muscles relaxed.

Leaving the church, I didn't expect a four-mile climb into a headwind. I finished the last mile of the climb at three miles per hour in the lowest gear before creeping over the 6,355-foot Continental Divide. I rode twenty more miles in the heaviest headwinds since last June in Wyoming. Before I had reached Lordsburg, rain started to pour. Soaking wet, I decided that forty-five miles for a short day wasn't bad—everything considered.

I awoke at five o'clock Monday morning with severe back pain. It was time to listen to my body and take the day off. I turned off the alarm, took two pain pills, and went back to sleep. Later, a leisurely breakfast was a rare luxury. As two loads of laundry tumbled through machines at a Laundromat, I wrote letters, reorganized the panniers, and removed three pounds of "nonessentials" to mail to Sharon. After cleaning, fine-tuning, and lubing the bike, I combined a check ride with a trip to the post office. A pleasant dinner with a glass of Chardonnay followed by a call to Elisabeth ended my "day off."

At four the next morning, I showered, did stretching exercises, loaded the bike, rode to El Charro Restaurant for breakfast, then headed west on I-10 at 5:55 A.M.

At this early hour I saw few autos but hundreds of semis. I watched the rearview mirror as they overtook me. About half signaled and moved into the left lane. The other half drilled down the outside lane as the blast of air from their rigs first blew me toward the embankment, then sucked me back toward the traffic in the following vacuum.

At first I felt their action was deliberate, as many touring cyclists believe. Motorcycle riders have told me they experience similar problems. It seems that many truckers have no idea of the havoc they create by coming so close. But after sharing more than 13,000 miles of America's roadways with drivers of the big rigs, I'm convinced most are considerate drivers. They just need to understand the problem, a problem serious enough to be discussed during truck driver training.

I turned south off I-10 onto U.S. 80 and stopped at Road Forks, New Mexico, where Shady Grove Restaurant and Truck Stop attracted my attention. Forty-seven Whites, Macks, Kenworths, Peterbilts, and other big rigs were in the parking lot. Inside, tasteful southwestern art and attractive hanging flowers adorned walls and ceiling of the restaurant where I devoured my second breakfast.

The nearby mall included a gift shop, CB radio shop, Radio Shack, laundry, post office, and the Professional Truckers Hall of Fame where technical information and the history of many makes of trucks was displayed. Pictures of truckers elected to the hall of fame and poems and essays written by and about truckers were on display.

Deciding to visit the American Museum of Natural History's Southwestern Research Station in the nearby Chiricahua Mountains, I turned west off U.S. 80. Seven miles later I was in Portal, Arizona.

A steep climb began at the mouth of Cave Creek Canyon where clear water tumbled from snowcapped peaks. Closer at hand, red rocks, covered by pale green and yellow lichens, contrasted with the green of pines, oaks, and junipers on lower slopes. Charming mountains, those Chiricahuas.

At Cathedral Vista Point, I locked Old Faithful to a tree and walked the nature trail where signs identified plants and described their uses. Some were old friends. Others, such as the short Chihuahua pine and the taller alligator juniper were new to me. Good to know the plants and animals of a place.

Returning to the road, I found a man surveying my loaded bicycle. Robert Waldmire was, he told me, a freelance poster artist. His Volkswagen bus was decorated with painted flowers and peace symbols. He lived only twenty-five miles from San Diego. "When you get that far west," he insisted, "you must stay with me so the last day of your journey will be short."

After reaching the station that evening, I had supper with staff, students, and scientists. They described their projects while showing me the laboratories and research library. Two javelina burst out of a dry wash, nearly running me down as I returned to my rustic cabin. These fascinating, piglike creatures added an exclamation point to day's end.

After emerging from the canyon, I returned to New Mexico only long enough to pick up a few supplies in the village of Rodeo, then rode back into Arizona, where I stopped at the Geronimo Surrenders Monument. The inscribed message told that Geronimo, the last Apache chief, surrendered on

September 6, 1886, to General Nelson A. Miles. Geronimo's surrender forever ended Indian warfare in the United States.

Highway repairs a few miles north of Douglas stopped traffic until a pilot car led a line of vehicles, mine included, over the construction area. After feeling lousy for so long, I enjoyed the incredulous looks from motorists and construction workers as I held my place in line at twenty-four miles per hour for two miles of newly blacktopped highway. Yes, it was slightly downhill.

That night I pitched my tent in the Douglas Camping and RV Park and enjoyed dinner at the Dawson Restaurant and Saloon.

🚲 🚲 🚲

A mountain near Bisbee, Arizona, appeared to have the top sheared off. It was the Lavender Pit, a huge copper ore excavation site. I lunched on a Monte Carlo sandwich at the Copper Queen Hotel, built in 1902 when Bisbee was the largest copper mining town in the world.

In the 1870s soldiers from Fort Huachuca discovered silver deposits while on patrol for "hostile Apaches" near the present site of Bisbee. It soon became evident that copper, not silver, was the dominant mineral. But during silver's fleeting fame, the Silver King Hotel was built in 1900 on Brewery Avenue, formerly Brewery Gulch. Bisbee's population was reduced to 15,000 by 1914, but there were still forty saloons in Brewery Gulch, many dance halls, and innumerable "dance hall girls." Wild, reckless, sometimes violent social life was still common. It was reported, however, that Brewery Gulch never had a skid row. Substantial stone and brick businesses and homes dominated lower portions of the gulch, though miners' homes on the steep slopes were only shacks.

Phelps Dodge Corporation began working the Sacramento Pit in 1917. This became the first open pit copper mine in Arizona. By 1929 the copper deposits were exhausted and, after 43 million tons of earth, rocks, and ore were removed, a huge crater occupied the landmark once called Sacramento Hill.

In April 1951 Phelps Dodge started work on another mountain near Bisbee. According to a brochure I read in Bisbee:

*The company spent 25 million dollars and three years to remove 46 million
tons of barren cappings and truck the earth and rocks to waste dumps*

before any ore was milled. As much as 350 feet of waste was removed in places before exposing ore. By December 1974 the ore was depleted, the mountain gone, and all mining operations closed by June 1975.

Rather cavalier language, I thought, to describe the destruction of a mountain.

I did find much charm in this elongated town as I climbed six miles from an elevation of 5,300 at the lower end of New Bisbee to 6,000 feet at the upper end of Old Bisbee. On advice of a cyclist, I took the old highway to avoid a dangerous tunnel on U.S. 80 before descending along the Mule Mountains toward Tombstone.

When the county seat of Cochise County was moved from Tombstone to Bisbee in 1930, objections were so vigorous that it required a decision by the Arizona Supreme Court. An editorial appeared in the *Tombstone Epitaph* saying "Let it be known that the spirit of Tombstone is to never say die." This was embellished to the town's now world-famous slogan "The Town Too Tough to Die."

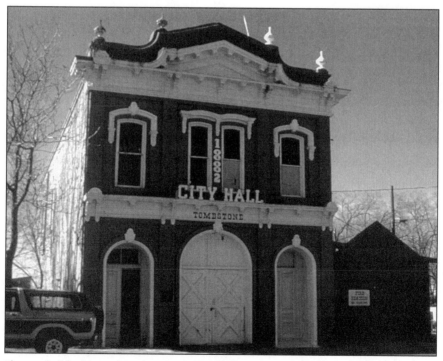

The city hall building of Tombstone, Arizona

Many western movies, books, and songs have their settings in Tombstone fact and lore, yet it is not a "stage-prop town." Sturdily built brick buildings have been maintained to look as they did in the 1880s. I never saw any western facades fronting modern buildings. Of course exaggerated stories of the whoring, drinking, gunfighting days in frontier Tombstone are carried out in such attractions as Boothill, O.K. Corral, Bird Cage Theatre, and Crystal Palace. Still, at the Silver Nugget Museum I was impressed to find solid documentation, in pictures and words, of those free-wheeling days.

Portrayed as Tombstone's most authentic attraction, the Bird Cage was described in 1882 by the *New York Times* as the "wildest, wickedest night life between Basin Street and the Barbary Coast."

During its nine-year life from 1881 to 1889, the Bird Cage lived up to its billing. The 140 bullet holes in walls and ceilings of the gambling casino, dance hall, and poker room are mute evidence of the sixteen gunfights reported during this period.

Stage entertainment ranged from nightly French circuit cancan dancers to risqué performances for men only to headliners such as Eddie Foy, Lotta Crabtree, and others. Under the stage is the poker room where the longest poker game in western history ran continuously for eight years, five months, and three days. It cost $1,000 in chips to buy into a game. The poker table still stands as it was left—with its chairs on the dirt floor.

The most publicized features were the fourteen Bird Cage Crib Compartments, still draped with red velvet and suspended from the ceiling over the gambling casino and dance hall. Here "ladies of the night" entertained their men friends, assisted by a red-coated bartender who placed drinks on a dumbwaiter for delivery "upstairs."

Following a night of back pain, I knew floor exercises were essential to a day of biking. Getting out of bed and prone on the floor was tough. After a few stretches, crunches, and attempted push-ups, I had one helluva time getting on my feet. Holding onto a chair and the bed, and using only arm strength, I stood upright only to collapse from severe muscle spasms. This happened twice before I was finally on my feet.

Tired and hurting after riding only twenty miles, I was beginning a climb when I met cyclist Tom Alinen. He turned and rode up beside me.

"Saw your heavy load and wondered where you were headed. Mind if I ride with you?"

Tom, a sergeant with the police department in Sierra Vista, was training for a fifty-mile ride. At first I resented having my misery interrupted, but Tom was such a friendly, interesting guy that I soon forgave him. A Vietnam veteran, he had taken intelligence training at Fort Huachuca and liked that area so much he returned after service. By the time we reached the top of the seven-mile climb, I was sweating but pleased at feeling little discomfort or fatigue.

With a "Well, I'd better get back home. Good luck on the rest of your trip," he was gone and so was my self-pity. I reflected that, though I preferred riding alone, there were advantages to companionship. Sometimes, I'd had too much time to examine my pain and fatigue while pounding out the miles alone.

🚲 🚲 🚲

Dr. George Post, a colleague at CSU, retired two years ahead of me and built an earth-sheltered home near Rio Rico. I had called from Douglas to tell him my planned route was fifty miles north of Rio Rico but I wanted to say hello while in the neighborhood. "Give me a call when you reach Sonoita," George said. "I'll pick you up and you can stay overnight with us."

While waiting in Sonoita, I went to the bank to get cash on my Visa card. For the first time on this trip, Visa declined payment. It took fifteen minutes of talking to the Visa people in California before the teller discovered the problem and obtained approval. In the meantime, I asked the banker if he could suggest a place to store my bike while I visited George and Charlotte. He mentioned a machine shop a half mile away. I was ready to pedal when he dashed out of the bank and said, "Just got to thinking. We'll be closing soon, but you can wheel your bike in here for the night. We open at nine in the morning. You can pick it up any time after that."

The Posts' home was spacious and well-adapted to the harsh desert environment. In the morning we visited Nogales and the international fence separating Nogales, Arizona, from Nogales, Mexico, a stark reminder of how we deal with our neighbors to the south.

🚲 🚲 🚲

Highlights of my stop in Tucson were the Mariachi singers at Saint Augustine's on Sixth Avenue, where I attended eight o'clock mass, and a brief visit with Seymour Levy whom I'd not seen since we graduated from the University of Idaho in 1949. He and his brother Jimmy had a taxidermy shop and guided bird hunters in the fall. Several years before my visit, they had been given the Arizona Conservationist of the Year Award. Two hours was a short time for lunch with Seymour and his wife, Helen, and to catch up on the past thirty-seven years.

After cycling to Gilbert Ray Campground, I awakened the next morning at 2:45 A.M. to hear coyotes serenading in such clear, full tones that I recorded their moonlit performance. Sandi, who transcribed my tapes back in Fort Collins, would appreciate a break from listening to me. At 4:30 A.M., two coyotes joined voices. I couldn't sleep so decided to enjoy the loud duet while striking camp and packing the bike by flashlight and moonlight. A few handfuls of trail mix and I was on my way at daybreak.

A sixtyish fellow enjoying the morning sun sat on a bench in front of the roadside cafe where I stopped for coffee. In response to my "Good morning," he quickly returned the greeting, said his name was "Angel," and expressed keen interest in my bike trip. He was one-fourth Hispanic, three-fourths Papago. He had lived nearby all his life. He said he was lonely and liked to say "Good morning" to people, but most either ignored him or looked at him as if he were just a drunken old Indian.

"You're the first tourist to say good morning to me in a long time," he said wistfully. I invited him to come in for coffee and a bite to eat.

When I ordered coffee and two pieces of hot apple pie, he said, "Oh, no, I'll just have coffee."

While I enjoyed the pie and coffee, Angel filled me in on the large Papago Reservation I would be entering in a few miles. "Where do you think you'll stay tonight?" he asked.

"I plan to make it to Sells."

"Don't know of a motel but I know a guy in Sells who might let you pitch your tent in his backyard. His name is Windy."

A fellow at the counter spoke up: "I'll bet you're talking about Earle Winderman. I've seen him and his white wolf dog at Old Tucson where they're making a western movie. They're bit players."

I called the Sells operator. Instead of giving me a phone number, she got Earle on the phone. "I'm an old retired professor on a year-long bike ride," I explained, not wanting him to think I was a hippie looking for a handout.

His immediate response was, "I'm a retired academic, too. Sure you can pitch your tent here. Plan to have dinner with us."

It was nearly dark when I rolled up to his home. Earle met me in the yard with, "Don't know what I was thinking when you asked about setting up your tent. You're staying in the house. I'll help unload your bike and get your gear inside." Earle, it turned out, was Dr. Winderman, a retired professor who moved from Pennsylvania to Arizona because his wife, Joan, needed a warm, dry climate for her health. Joan taught reading skills to Papago children. The dog recalled by the fellow in the cafe was three-fourths wolf. It was beautiful and seemed perfectly disciplined.

Dinner featured wine, salad, soup, and a delicious chicken dish—a welcome change from energy bars and restaurant food. Two young Papago men came by. It was obvious they looked to the Windermans as mentors and friends. Conversation turned to an article in the morning's *Arizona Daily Star* headlined "New O'odham law elicits fear, confusion."

According to the article, the adoption of a new tribal constitution in a special election six weeks before my arrival was of concern to many tribal members. Some felt the voters were apathetic and inadequately informed. Others were concerned because the constitution replaced the old name of Papago with Tohono O'odham, or "Desert People."

After crossing eighty-seven miles of mostly barren landscape in this 2.8 million-acre reservation, I had seen the deep poverty and lack of employment opportunity and could guess why apathy and suicide were major problems here. I was ashamed my government had assigned this land they didn't want as the Papagos' homeland.

🚲 🚲 🚲

The next post office where I had arranged a mail pickup was in Why, just west of the reservation. Hearing that their post office opened only a few hours daily, I decided to find what time I would have to be in town to pick up mail. No telephone was listed for the Why post office, so I called the next town, Ajo.

The postmistress there said the Why post office opened only from ten to two. It was unlikely I could make it before they closed. The lady in Ajo solved my dilemma with, "I know the postmistress in Why. I'll call her at home and ask her to send your mail here in the morning."

"I may not get to Ajo before you close," I said.

"If you are late just come around and knock on the side door. Ask for Annette and I'll get your mail for you."

Arriving an hour after closing the next evening, I knocked at the side door. Annette cheerfully brought out the mail along with directions to "the best restaurant in town."

I had biked several blocks when a pickup passed and pulled over. Annette jumped out. "I got to thinking about my directions and realized I'd forgotten about an important turn. I figured I could catch you before you got lost."

正 正 正

At the Gatlin Site, three miles north of Gila Bend, a 1,000-year-old Hohokam Indian village was being excavated and studied. As many as 200 Hohokams lived there between A.D. 900 and 1,100. Anthropologists and archaeologists believe the Hohokam population in the Southwest desert may have reached 50,000. They were successful farmers who constructed the first major irrigation system on the North American continent.

Internationally prominent ecologist and ethnobotanist Gary Paul Nabhan in his widely acclaimed book, *Gathering the Desert,* points out that in areas with only three to twelve inches of rainfall annually, native Indians, even without irrigation, had developed a remarkable agricultural civilization. Nabhan warns that, "Irrevocable groundwater depletion in arid zones is becoming a common tragedy." He believes that employing agricultural practices of early Indian tribes and planting their ancient grains, many with outstanding nutritional qualities, not only helps Indians save their traditional agriculture, but may point a way to overcoming agricultural problems caused by a rapidly diminishing supply of water.

Nabhan found that people often think of deserts as wastelands, not recognizing the value of wild plants, historic crops, and traditions of Indian farming in maintaining sustainable food production on this harsh land.

Leaving Gila Bend, I would follow I-8, more or less, until reaching San Diego, now only 300 miles away. Despite late-day headwinds, I rode seventy-five miles to Tacna. One of my longer days recently and I felt good about it.

The next day I-8 rose steeply toward a pass. To avoid a long climb, I decided to make an end run around the Gila Mountains by taking the old highway along the Gila River as it followed a horseshoe bend known as Dome Valley. The barren desert gave way to fertile, irrigated fields as I entered the valley. Crops of lettuce and onions and groves of orange and grapefruit trees marched away from the highway in orderly rows. A sign announced the McClenney Cattle Ranch with 90,000 head of beef cattle.

I took a dozen photos of the neatness and straight lines of the row crops, and the photogenic symmetry of the orchards. In addition to crops seen earlier, I noted rows of cauliflower, broccoli, and radishes. There were fields of cotton and alfalfa.

I talked with several Anglo farmers and business people. Despite evidence of prosperity, piecework wages were low and living quarters for the undocumented workers who supplied the "stoop labor" to plant, cultivate, and harvest the crops were shoddy. Lack of education opportunities for the workers' children and need for medical services and better housing for the families were obvious.

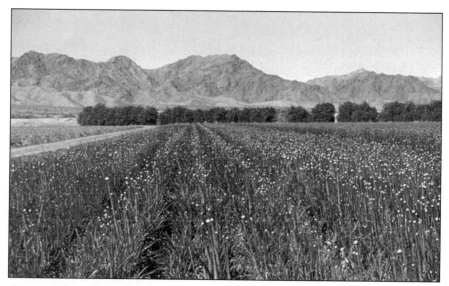

Onions grow in the irrigated fields of Dome Valley along the Gila River.

Yuma, an aggressively booming city, dates its modern beginning to 1850 when California gold-seekers learned that the "Yuma Crossing" was one of the better sites to cross the Colorado River. Yuma grew slowly at first. A spurt of growth after World War II brought the population in 1950 to 9,145. The current estimate is more than 100,000.

My Saturday morning reconnaissance of the city led to the North End, a restoration project where they were celebrating citizen participation. Seven hours of foot and bike races were underway, but scents and sights at the Garden Cafe and Spice Company captured my attention. An imaginative omelet, with fresh fruit and gourmet coffee, was served on a terraced patio surrounded by palms, orange trees, and an aviary separated from the dining area only by a light netting. The cockatoos, doves, and a variety of songbirds added a pleasant profusion of color and sound.

I talked with several people while watching the races. A seventy-year-old man, tan and in superb condition, exuded enthusiasm as he told of his bicycling, running, and swimming activities. The year before he had been the oldest finisher in the Ironman Triathlon in Hawaii. A few months after that, he ran 101 miles in a twenty-four-hour period.

Back at the motel in Yuma, I asked the desk clerk if there was a good breakfast place in Waterhaven, California. "If I were riding a bicycle, I wouldn't stop there," he replied.

"Why not?"

"I just don't like that place. A lot of bad things happen."

"Like what?"

"It's just a bad place. I don't think you should stop there for breakfast. OK?"

Ignoring the warning, I stopped in Winterhaven at a small, definitely blue-collar cafe for a short stack and coffee. The boisterous talk and good-natured kidding among workers reminded me of logging and construction camps where I'd worked. I felt right at home.

Shortly after turning onto State Highway 98 at the Gordon Wells exit, I noticed a large canal closely paralleling the highway. My map showed it was only a few hundred yards from the Mexico border.

A few miles later, on a straight stretch about ten miles east of Calexico, I noticed a fellow with a backpack and bag climbing up the bank onto the highway about a hundred yards ahead. He was followed by another fellow, then another, all with packs and bags. They looked my way, hesitated a moment, then dropped their bags, grabbed hands, and stretched across the highway. By this time, I was about seventy-five feet away. Not a good situation.

I don't remember forming any strategy. I just kicked in full power and headed straight toward the man stretching toward the shoulder I was riding. He, and the other two, began yelling in Spanish. I do recall thinking I could swerve at the last moment, miss the guy, and still not go over the embankment. Fortunately, that wasn't necessary. I was looking straight at the fellow and saw disbelief in his eyes just as I steeled myself to swerve. Falling back, he let out a huge bellow and his outflung hand brushed my shoulder as I zipped by at twenty-five miles per hour. I'd won the game of "Chicken" and received a shot of adrenalin as well. Westward ho!

In Calexico I called Sharon to tell her that I would be in San Diego in a couple of days. She surprised me with, "Dad, call me when you reach San Diego. I will book the next flight out of Aspen. Gary and I were with you when you began your adventure. I want to be there when you finish. We can fly back to Colorado together."

That night, I slept well and arose ready to challenge two significant climbs between Calexico and the coast. The first was a long climb where a cyclist in Yuma had said I might have to get off and push. I was pleased to climb 3,200 feet in eight miles, a 7.5 percent grade, without dismounting.

A final serious climb brought me from Jacumba, elevation 2,850, to Tecate Divide at 4,118 feet. Here, I photographed sixteen wind turbines. According to the American Wind Energy Association, California began building wind farms in 1981 with 144 small turbines generating seven megawatts of electricity. By the end of 1985 that had grown to 12,391 turbines and 1,007 megawatts, enough electricity to service a city of over 300,000 people.

The advantages of this power source are obvious. It doesn't require precious water resources and, except for visual impact and noise, doesn't degrade the environment nor deplete limited resources as do coal-fired plants. Nor does it present the dangers of nuclear power plants. In the long run, it is more economical. Why, then, has wind power developed so slowly? It is largely because the American public is not very good at thinking in the long term and even worse at paying up front to protect the environment.

In Alpine I dialed the number Bob Waldmire, the artist I had met in the Chirachaua Mountains, had told me to call from Alpine. I was directed down Harbison Canyon to where I would see a large "Swallows Sun Island" sign. I wondered if Bob lived at an artist's colony or camp or what. In a few miles a solid redwood fence about eight feet high displayed the sign beside a solid wood gate the same height. A sign directed me to press a button. A small panel slid open, revealing a pair of eyes, and a female voice asked, "Are you Dwight Smith?"

My identity established, the gate swung open. "Welcome to Swallows," said friendly Sue Latimer, co-owner of Swallows. Several people, in various stages of undress, were walking about in open areas of what looked like an RV Park. I soon discovered this was a family-oriented nudist resort. When Bob was located, he suggested I pitch my tent on a grassy area, stow my sleeping bag and gear inside, and accompany him on a walking tour.

Some residents lived in modest homes built since Sun Island's beginning in 1954, others in mobile homes. Motor homes and a small motel were occupied mostly by "snowbird nudists" or other nonresident nudists. There were about 100 permanent residents, many retired. Younger couples with children from toddlers to teenagers lived there, too. Many had jobs in San Diego and surrounding communities.

Recreational facilities included a swimming pool, tennis courts, and ping-pong tables. The youth center was called "Nude-Niks Nest." That sign was the only photo I took inside the resort. Bob said to feel free to photograph anything or anybody. But I would have felt like an old lecher to go around snapping pix of bare boobs and buns, though he assured me nothing was off-limits.

We had dinner at the community dining room. Many residents prepared meals in their own abodes; others preferred the communal setting. The plain but clean dining room featured long picniclike tables with benches for seating. A few diners were completely clothed, others buck naked. Bob's only garb was a red bandanna tied around his head. Some wore only T-shirts, others only shorts.

Friendly, lighthearted conversation flowed as in a large family. Bob introduced me to everyone close by. One portly lady advised taking advantage of their outdoor Jacuzzi. "It will relax you for a good night's sleep so you'll be rested for your last day of biking."

I walked to the brightly lit, fenced-in Jacuzzi at eight o'clock. A sign on the gate ordered "No Bathing Suits Allowed." Six men, three women, and two little girls were in the water. More came later. I was more at ease than I had expected. It was the first time I had experienced nudism since skinny-dipping in the creek as a kid.

Friendly conversation continued and I was immediately included. Les and his wife, Ginni, were avid cyclists and runners. Les went to his house for a San Diego map, then marked a route to the Adams Avenue Bicycle Shop where I had called to ask them to pack my bike for the flight to Fort Collins.

Just before six o'clock the next morning, it was cold enough that I wore long biking pants and a jacket while striking camp and packing the bike.

A shuffling sound on the dirt road caused me to look up. A man walking past wore nothing but sandals, a sweatshirt over his torso, a wool cap pulled over his ears, and a huge smile. I had to suppress outright laughter. Soon he came back with the morning paper and called out, "Have a good ride. Glad you visited us. Come back again."

The twenty miles to the edge of San Diego where I stopped for coffee and a doughnut passed quickly. Leaving The Donut Shop, I soon became lost. The street sign at a major intersection where Les had told me to turn made no sense at all. While I puzzled over the map, a bicyclist rode up beside me. "May I help you?"

"According to this map I should turn here, but this street sign isn't the same as on the map," I grumbled. He looked at the sign, then snorted, "Some clown turned the sign ninety degrees. They're always doing that around here. But you're headed the right way."

After a couple of miles I came to a place where Les, in the nudist colony Jacuzzi, had suggested taking a bike trail to avoid heavy traffic. "It's a little tricky to find the trail," he had warned. After turning onto the trail entrance, I was rechecking the map when a UPS truck pulled up and the driver asked if I was planning to take that trail. When I responded, "Yes," he continued, "I watched you horse that load up this hill and didn't want to see you ride an extra two miles for nothing. Last week they started trail repairs. In a mile you would find a 'Trail Closed' sign and have to come back." With that he made a U-turn and headed back down the hill. Open-mouthed, I realized he had driven up just to save me some fruitless riding.

One more Good Samaritan helped me to negotiate the last mile. A cyclist came up fast, then slowed beside me. "Where are you heading?" he asked.

"Adams Avenue Bicycle Shop."

"That's just a mile ahead, but it's hard to see from this direction. Traffic is too heavy for me to ride beside you so I'll ride behind and yell when you should turn off."

When he shouted, "Turn here, you're going past it!" I responded with a grateful "Thank you" and soon stopped in front of the bike shop. It was March 18, 1986. The odometer recorded 13,784 miles. Old Faithful and I were both a little worse for wear, but we had done it. The circle had been closed.

CHAPTER FIFTEEN

After the Ride

Only that traveling is good which reveals to me the value
of home, and enables me to enjoy it better.

—Henry David Thoreau

Home again in Fort Collins, at first I missed the routine of getting up at dawn, loading Old Faithful, and heading into a new day, not knowing what to expect but anticipating some new adventure. Soon, though, new routines took over. An early task was to complete reviewing and editing the 1,900 pages transcribed from my taped journal and to finish cataloging the 2,500 photos taken.

The Colorado State University team of specialists reassembled in July to repeat the same battery of tests conducted in 1984 so we could compare my physical condition before and after the trip. Dr. Loren Cordain, professor of exercise and sport science, then compared my results with those in studies at the University of Louisville and by Dr. Ken Cooper on the relationship of aerobic capacity and cholesterol with age. In both cases, aerobic capacity decreased with age with the decline most rapid after age fifty, and cholesterol increased with age and decreased with exercise.

My aerobic capacity, instead of declining at age sixty-four, had increased substantially in the twenty-six months between the pre- and post-trip measurements. After the trip my aerobic capacity was 36 percent higher than the average for a fifty-two-year-old group in the Louisville study, and my cholesterol level had declined to 169, well below the average of 185 for that group.

Cardiovascular effects in terms of heart rate and blood pressure were tested on a bicycle ergometer. Nine minutes of strenuous exercise raised my heart rate to 172 beats per minute in 1984. After two minutes recovery it dropped to 161 and to 121 after five minutes. In the same test in 1986 my heart rate rose only to 160, then dropped to 120 and 105 after two and five minutes, respectively.

Blood pressure after nine minutes of exercise read 200/98 in 1984, and 192/98 in 1986. After a three-minute recovery period in 1984, blood pressure was 178/94; in 1986 it was 164/80, a far more rapid recovery than before the bike ride. Handgrip strength increased an average of 16.4 percent during the ride.

After reviewing results of these tests, Dr. Cordain concluded that my lungs, heart, and muscles had improved markedly at an age when they would normally decline.

My results thus follow those of others. Reese Walton first rode in the El Tour de Tucson bicycle race when sixty-five, finishing the 111-mile event in seven hours, forty-nine minutes. Seven years later his time was only seven hours, seven minutes. At age seventy-seven, he rode the 111 miles in seven hours and forty-one minutes, still eight minutes faster than at age sixty-five. Also when seventy-seven, he pedaled the grueling 252-mile Cochise County Classis in eighteen hours! When interviewed by *Tailwinds* three years later, Reese remarked, "I am eighty years old but I feel joyous about my life and my age. I'm grateful I can still cycle competitively."

The same issue of *Tailwinds* reported that eighty-two-year-old Gordy Shields had completed the 111-mile event in the remarkable time of seven hours, two minutes. Afterward he said, "I may have a little bursitis, some carpal tunnel, a twitch in my spine, but none of that affects my ability to ride. And cycling offers a camaraderie in which age doesn't matter."

USA Today carried a story of Jim Tatum, seventy-six, whose four-man relay team, all over the age of seventy, bicycled from the Pacific Coast in California to the Atlantic Coast in Georgia in eight days, nine hours, and eleven minutes. When asked how he felt about old age, Jim retorted, "When I get there, I'll tell you!" The same issue told of Earl Shaffer, seventy-nine, who had hiked the 2,160-mile Appalachian Trail, and Lenny Aikins, who still parachuted six times a week at age eighty-three.

Rocky Mountain Sports reported that in thirty-seven years, Bob Martin had climbed 5,040 peaks, including all fifty-five peaks in Colorado over 14,000 feet. At age eighty, Bob still had a schedule of peaks to climb.

Cole Kugel, the oldest certified pilot in America, flew until he was ninety-nine. His wife died in June 2001 after they had flown together for more than a half century. Before her death she told Cole, "Don't you sell that plane until I'm gone." A few months after she died, he finally sold their old Cessna with the stipulation that he could take it up on his 100th birthday.

The *Fort Collins Coloradoan* reported that Norman Vaughan had accompanied Admiral Byrd to Antarctica in 1928 and returned sixty-six years later at age eighty-nine to climb 10,302-foot Mount Vaughan, which Byrd had named for him. When interviewed Vaughan said, "People should look forward to retirement but not think of it in terms of an armchair."

These examples show that seniors are truly capable of much more than we think. Although many folks over sixty envied my bicycle journey, they dismissed such an adventure for themselves because they said they were "too old." I can only agree with Joe Friel who, in his carefully documented *Cycling Past 50*, concluded that much of our "slowing down" stems from inactivity and other self-imposed limitations rather than physiological losses.

ᘓᕓ ᘓᕓ ᘓᕓ

Elisabeth sold her home in Michigan in 1987 and bought a small home in Fort Collins. We biked and hiked together, joined a square dance club, and in early autumn drove to California where we cycled 400 miles through the redwoods. But a year later I was diagnosed with an unpleasant form of arthritis and although we continued biking, hiking, and dancing, these activities became more and more difficult for me. Eventually our relationship began to fall off. We remained good friends, though, meeting occasionally on the bike trails.

Prednisone, anti-inflammatory drugs, and increasingly vigorous exercise brought gradual improvement, and in 1991 I returned to serious cycling when the 111-mile El Tour de Tucson, an annual event attracting some 4,000 cyclists, was dedicated to me. I was the last to finish. But I *did* finish!

My flying increased and my daughter Sharon and son, Gary, flew with me when they could. On a memorable sixteen-day flying/camping adventure to Alaska, Sharon and I alternated in flying the plane. On our return to Colorado, foul weather forced us to make two emergency landings in the Yukon, one piloted by Sharon and one by me. We had kept our own pilot log book and it was fun to discover that we each had logged exactly 34.3 hours as pilots!

In 1994 I met Yvonne, widow of a Vietnam veteran, on a hike to the cabin from where I had filmed for a television documentary twenty-three years earlier. The steep, rocky trail began at 9,000 feet and took us over the Continental Divide at 12,100 feet. After scrambling down the other side to the cabin at timberline, we climbed back over the divide and returned to the trailhead. It was a tough one-day hike, but Yvonne's determination and obvious fascination with the rugged mountains captured me.

Later, though she had never before flown in a small plane, Yvonne began flying with me. No wonder I fell in love with her!

With Yvonne as an enthusiastic companion, I set new goals. She started riding with me on day-rides and various cycling events, including El Tour de Tucson. Later she wisely convinced me that the fifty-mile option, rather than the 111-mile event, would be more fun and leave us with more energy afterward. Soon we were skiing and square dancing together too.

By the spring of 1997 I needed some quiet time for reading, reflecting, and writing. We arranged to spend a year at Desert House of Prayer in Tucson as part-time retreatants and part-time volunteer staff.

We were just settled at Desert House when news came that Elisabeth had entered the Fort Collins hospital for knee surgery. Internal bleeding and a hepatic aneurysm followed and she had died. Yvonne had met Elisabeth at square dances and on bike trails and liked her. We grieved her death together.

After ten months at Desert House, "part-time staff" was requiring more and more time so we returned to Fort Collins to finish the book. Other interests, however, continued to interfere with writing. I had ridden in thirty-four states so, with Yvonne as a delightful companion, I cycled in the remaining sixteen to achieve another goal—to ride in all fifty states.

Failing eyesight and hearing finally forced me to abandon my plan to also pilot a small plane in all fifty states. I settled, instead, for twenty-six states and hundreds of splendid memories. But, needing motivation to keep physically active, I soon added another target. On my seventy-eighth birthday Yvonne and I bicycled seventy-eight miles, beginning what we hoped would become our annual gift of health and happiness to each other for years to come.

Epilogue

I had left Fort Collins on my journey not at all certain that I would return. Although I loved the mountains and climate, the triple tragedies of losing Alan, Mark, and Carol often brought painful memories in these familiar surroundings.

Biases I had not recognized rode with me as I began this journey. From the piney woods of Georgia, through Florida, Alabama, and Mississippi to the swamplands of Louisiana, I often biked through rural areas, small communities, and big-city neighborhoods populated entirely or mostly by blacks. This was new to me, and though I was never once threatened, I often felt uneasy. The fact was that on several occasions, friendly blacks helped where others ignored my needs.

Similar experiences unfolded from Esperanza, Texas, to Caballo, New Mexico, as I wended my sometimes apprehensive way along the Rio Grande. Yet people in those predominantly Mexican communities were friendly and helpful.

Unexpected kindness and uncommon generosity were extended in big cities from the boroughs of New York City to the coastal areas of Los Angeles.

Over the years, I had visited most of these areas except for rural areas in the South. But those visits by auto or air were usually quick, casual, and often with companions. When experienced slowly and intimately from the seat of a bicycle, they brought very different impressions. Places I thought I had known now became new and fascinating environments and caused me to revise my opinions of places and people and to learn from our differences.

Considering these experiences, it seemed paradoxical that people often asked why I didn't carry a gun or warned me about dangerous people and communities ahead, revealing their distrust and fear of others. Only once was I threatened directly, and numerous near misses by speeding or crowding vehicles quickly taught that my mission was far more dangerous than I had anticipated. Had I surrendered to fear, however, this trip would not have been completed.

A review of my taped journal revealed that I also had begun the trip with an attitude that evolved through several stages before the journey ended. My determination to ride the perimeter of the United States quickly escalated into an attitude of belligerence toward other users of the road who crowded me or otherwise invaded my safety zone. No S.O.B. was going to stop me from completing this journey! That such belligerence had exposed me to unnecessary risks became apparent when I realized that I had had five accidents in the first 4,000 miles and none in the remaining 10,000.

Some of this improvement resulted from increased cycling skills, but more came from becoming less belligerent and simply riding assertively. This meant clearly signaling my intentions to motorists, then acting without hesitation. Though scary at first, this was the safest thing to do.

Many had pointed out to me the dangers of cycling on roadways where vehicles were hurtling past at seventy-five miles per hour. "You just don't have much control over your own safety," some said. After riding thousands of miles I accepted that I never had full control anyway, but that I could do my best then "let go ... and let God."

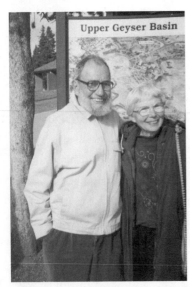

Upper Geyser Basin

This final attitude of acceptance pulled me toward my goal of finishing. Sometimes, too, it helped just to shout aloud my old lumberjack dad's admonishment years ago when I had thought I could do no more: "Hell, kid, I thought you hired out to be tough!"

Now, years later, I realize that this bicycle trip began as a way to honor my wife and two sons but became an ongoing journey to honor myself as well. My rough edges have softened and the gift of time has let me look deep within myself and become renewed.

As this book goes to press, I live in Fort Collins again and still bicycle for commuting, recreation, and staying in shape. And I can now look squarely at what I learned in those two years as Yvonne and I, together, look forward to the adventures and challenges of each new day.

As this book goes to press, Yvonne and I, together at ages sixty-four and eighty-two, look forward to the adventures and challenges of each new day. (Photo taken in Yellowstone National Park on September 18, 2003.)